THE ULTIM... ....
LOSE WEIGHT &
IMPROVE YOUR LIFE IN
2021: 3 BOOKS IN 1.
Keto Chaffle, Atkins Diet
& Renal Diet.
350+ Easy & Quick
Recipes to Fulfill Your
Family's Needs

AUTHOR
CHARLOTTE
CONLAN

KETO CHAFFLE COOKBOOK 2020-2021:

Two Years of Simple, Irresistible and Fast Low-Carb and Gluten Free Ketogenic Waffle Recipes – A Step-by-Step Guide to Lose and Maintain your Weight.

AUTHOR

CHARLOTTE CONLAN

TABLE OF CONTENTS

WHAT IS KETO DIET

The Ketogenic Diet is an uncommon diet high in fat, low in carbohydrate and moderate in protein, deliberately controlled. "Ketogenic" implies that a synthetic substance, called ketones, is delivered in the body.

The perfect Ketogenic Diet called the "long-chain triglyceride diet," gives 3 to 4 grams of fat for each gram of starch and protein. The "proportion" in the Ketogenic Diet is the proportion of fat for every gram of carbohydrate and protein joined. The kind of fat source foods of the Ketogenic Diet is margarine, cream or cream, mayonnaise, and oils.

Albeit the two carbohydrate and proteins in the diet are confined, it is basic to give enough measures of protein. It is likewise basic to set up the Ketogenic Diet painstakingly regulated by a Nutritionist, who observed the nutrition of the youngsters.

How Does The Keto Diet Work?

Generally, the body utilizes carbohydrate (sugar, bread, or pasta) as its fuel, yet in the Ketogenic Diet, the fat turns into the essential fuel. Ketones are one of the potential instruments of activity of the diet. There are various speculations, for example, the adjustment of glucose, adenosine, polyunsaturated unsaturated fats, and then some.

For Whom Is The Keto Diet Appropriate?

It is recommended for youngsters with seizures that are hard-headed to treatment. That is, they don't react to a few diverse anticonvulsant prescriptions. They have been utilized first in quite a while. Be that as it may, it is especially recommended for kids with Lennox-Gastaut disorder.

It is additionally reasonable for particular sorts of seizures or epileptic disorders, being valuable for myoclonic epilepsy of youth (Dravet disorder), asthmatic myoclonic epilepsy (Doose disorder), puerile fits (West disorder), mitochondrial abandons, Tuberous sclerosis complex (TSC), Rett disorder. Furthermore, for the GLUT 1 insufficiency disorder (GLUT1 DS) and pyruvate dehydrogenase inadequacy (PDH).

TYPES OF KETOGENIC DIET

"Diet" signifies various things to various individuals. It can mean the sorts of foods an individual routinely eats. Moreover, it can mean an extraordinary course of food/food limitations either for weight reduction or clinical purposes.

Be that as it may, in the keto-world, diet implies both.

The ketogenic diet can be either a perpetual method for eating or a transitory health improvement plan. In any case, every individual's needs and objectives for utilizing this diet ought to be considered throughout the whole procedure.

STANDARD KETOGENIC DIET (SKD)

The proportion for the SKD rendition is regularly 5% carbs, 75% fat, and 20% protein. The numbers for fat and protein may move a bit. Be that as it may, generally, fat is a tremendous piece of the diet and caloric admission.

This very well known form uses this simple idea: basically remain at or underneath carb utmost to stay in ketosis.

HIGH PROTEIN KETOGENIC DIET

Right now, it is accomplished similarly as in the standard ketogenic diet. An ordinary macronutrient proportion may look like 55-60% fat, 35-40% protein, and still 5% carbs. Similarly, as with the SKD, one must stay at or underneath as far as possible for ketosis to do something amazing.

TARGETED KETOGENIC DIET (TKD)

Have you ever known about carb-stacking before an exercise? This is the principle thought with the focus on a ketogenic diet.

In this way, around 30-an hour prior to work out, eat somewhere in the range of 25-50g of effectively edible carbs. The genuine number will rely upon the person's needs and the sort of exercise to be performed.

The better kind of carbs for this keto rendition is glucose-based food. The body utilizes glucose-based food more proficiently than fructose-based food. To explain, glucose-based food is generally scorched totally without tossing the body out of ketosis.

At last, post-exercise meals ought to incorporate a lot of protein and less fat. In the typical keto circumstance, fat is supported. Nonetheless, for muscle recuperation and supplement retention, protein is a superior decision for the focus on the ketogenic diet.

CYCLICAL KETOGENIC DIET (CKD)

This one sounds weird, thinking about what we've been realizing. CKD is for weight lifters and competitors who wish to manufacture fit bulk and still boost fat misfortune.

Right now, keep a standard keto diet for five days. At that point, you cycle into the two-day period of carb-stacking.

As far as possible on the first carb-stacking day will be 50g. On the second carb-stacking day, the carb tally will be somewhere in the range of 400-600g. The reason is to stack up on carbs, so the body is appropriately energized for the following five days of tiring exercises.

Significantly, CKD carb stacking ought not to be utilized as a "cheat day" for those utilizing the standard ketogenic diet. This methodology is appropriate just for incredibly dynamic people.

RESTRICTED KETOGENIC DIET

Right now, both carbs and calories are restricted. Clinical experts, for the most part, direct this rendition. This form might be valuable in malignant growth treatment. In light of studies, disease cells can't utilize ketones for energy and actually can starve to death.

Likewise, with any diet routine or way of life change, you should look for the guidance of a proper clinical expert before starting. Such experts will think about the individual's clinical history and current condition of health, just as individual needs and objectives.

HEALTH BENEFITS OF THE KETO DIET

People normally combine the ketogenic diet with fast weight reduction. In any case, that is not where it got its beginning. Also, it's absolutely not the stopping point undoubtedly.

There's no denying that weight reduction alone guides in the advancement of by and large health. What's more, with weight reduction comes to a large number of other cardiovascular and stomach related enhancements.

Not with standing, the rundown doesn't verge on halting there. We should take a gander at some different circumstances where this inconceivable method for eating has a constructive outcome.

EPILEPTIC SEIZURES

Initially, clinical experts built up the ketogenic diet to treat epilepsy in youngsters impervious to different prescriptions. In a 1920s report, Dr Russell Wilder saw a 90%

abatement in seizures in around 30% of subjects.

As one would expect, there was a huge drop in the number of patients staying in the examination. In any case, the outcomes were predictable with the rest of the subjects at the 3-month, half-year, and one-year interims.

Later information has discovered a half decrease in seizures in an assessment of very nearly 20 examinations with 1084 patients. Both with and without the utilization of anticonvulsant prescriptions, the ketogenic diet has been compelling in seizure decrease.

In light of the extraordinary outcomes in epilepsy patients, more research has been in progress. Reassuringly, it is indicating promising outcomes in the treatment of Alzheimer's Disease and Parkinson's Disease. The investigations demonstrate expanded insight and upgraded memory.

Essentially, fit as a fiddle, people notice more noteworthy mental lucidity, expanded capacity to center, just as better headache control. The "why" isn't totally clear now.

CORONARY ILLNESS PREVENTION

Almost certainly, a large portion of us understands that weight reduction assists lower with blooding pressure. Furthermore, cholesterol levels additionally improve from along these lines of eating. The ketogenic diet advances a high-fat (healthy fat) routine with restricted sugars. This brings down triglycerides and expands HDLs (great cholesterol).

This appears to be insane from the start since everyone lets us know "fat" is terrible. What's more, specialists have been instructing patients for a considerable length of time to eat a low-fat, heart-healthy diet. In any case, in opposition to that hypothesis, carbohydrate, not fat, are really a huge main impetus behind expanded triglycerides.

POLYCYSTIC OVARY SYNDROME

Polycystic ovary disorder accompanies fluctuated side effects. These incorporate skin break out, state of mind swings, barrenness, exhaustion, skin labels, and hair development on the chest, face, back, and toes. It likewise causes excruciating and sporadic menstrual cycles. Moreover, most of those influenced by PCOS experience weight put on or issues shedding pounds.

In what manner can the ketogenic diet help PCOS? It's all hormonal. Expanded measures of the hormones insulin and androgen are the necessary team for a PCOS finding.

With the ketogenic diet, glucose levels go down as ketone levels go up. Lower glucose levels mean lower insulin levels. Thus, this implies the ovaries have no compelling reason to deliver more androgens, the male hormone. The outcome is the decrease or annihilation of PCOS indications, including fruitlessness. Gotta love that!

DIMINISHED INFLAMMATION ISSUES.

This classification incorporates joint inflammation, bad-tempered gut disorder (IBS), skin breakout, and other skin issues. Fortunately for individuals with these issues, the ketogenic diet is essentially calming.

There are various kinds of ketones present in a nutritional ketosis state. One of these smothers an irritation particle usually found in incendiary procedures. In light of this marvelous connection between the ketogenic diet and incendiary help, more research is prospective.

GASTROINTESTINAL PROBLEMS

There is incredible news for people with gastrointestinal issues, for example, gas, swelling, indigestion, and heartburn. Grains, especially wheat, rye, and grain, are a food stick helping the grain hold its shape. The ketogenic diet is a without grain method for eating. In this way, these side effects ought to reduce or totally decrease just by following the plan.

Another guilty party for stomach and stomach related problems is sugary foods. Since the ketogenic diet's primary idea is low-carb, sugars won't be an issue for the belly either.

KETO CHAFFLES

What is Chaffle?

Waffles are typically made of a flour-based player. However, a chaffle is sans flour! Rather, chaffless are made of eggs and cheddar. I realize it sounds odd. However, it really works! What's more, dieters wherever are going insane for this new low-carb waffle hack.

Chaffless is an extraordinary path for those on the keto diet to get their waffle fix. They're additionally an incredible method to eat fewer carbs while as yet eating what you need! Regardless of whether it is a changed adaptation. There are additionally unlimited mixes for what you can add to it and how you can spruce up and use chaffless.

The basic formula for a chaffle contains cheddar, almond flour, and an egg. You combine the ingredients in a bowl and pour it on your waffle producer. Waffle creators are most likely on the ascent right now after this chaffle formula detonated a day or two ago prior. I was somewhat doubtful from the outset thinking there was no chance this would turn out in the wake of combining everything and pouring the hitter on the waffle. I was expecting one enormous major chaos. Try to shower the waffle producer truly well. The waffle ended up extraordinary, and it was firm outwardly and delicate in the centre.

Step by step instructions to make chaffles

The main bit of kitchen hardware you have to make these keto chaffles is a waffle producer. I've made chaffles effectively in an ordinary size Belgian waffle producer. What's more, I've made littler size chaffles in a small waffle creator. I like the littler size better for chaffle sandwiches.

It appears as though individuals are having the most achievement utilizing this Dash Mini Waffle Iron. It is the ideal size to Cook them rapidly. Also, the littler size aides the chaffles fresh up perfectly.

My main tip for making crispier chaffles is to utilize a smaller than usual waffle creator like the Dash. I believe that this small scale waffle creator has the best volume to surface territory proportion to give you the crispiest outcomes.

Another tip is to ensure you to cook the chaffles sufficiently long. For me, it takes around 4 minutes for each chaffle to get brilliant dark colored. They may be somewhat delicate when you first expel them from the waffle creator, yet they will fresh up additional as they cool.

A third tip is to sprinkle some additional cheddar on the chaffle hitter part of the way through Cooking. The cheddar will liquefy and fresh up to make the chaffles extra firm.

You can likewise freeze chaffles. One extraordinary approach to meal Prep is to make a major bunch of chaffles and freeze them to eat later.

To freeze chaffles, freeze them on a Preparing sheet in a solitary layer (so they don't stay together). When they are solidified, place them in a cooler sack with a bit of material paper between each.

In the event that you don't have the cooler space to fit an entire heating sheet, you can freeze them in a cooler sack with a bit of material paper isolating them.

To serve, you can warm them in the microwave for 2-3 minutes. On the off chance that you have additional time, you can warm in a 350F stove or air fryer for crispier outcomes.

You can add a wide range of flavourings to plain chaffle hitter to make new kinds of chaffles.

- Try exploring different avenues regarding various types of cheddar. Cheddar is the first flavour, yet in addition use Monterrey Jack, Colby, mozzarella cheddar, and so on. You could even consolidate two various types of cheddar for included flavour — like a blend of mozzarella and Parmesan for a seasoned Italian Chaffle.

- Add flavours, for example, garlic powder, Italian flavouring, everything except the Bagel flavouring, or arranged herbs.

- Experiment with including keto-accommodating fruits and vegetables to your chaffle hitter. Think little solidified blueberries, or finely hacked peppers and onions.

- For much lighter chaffles, you can include a teaspoon of coconut flour or a tablespoon of almond flour to the egg blend. For a definitive fluffiest chaffles, include 1/4 tsp Preparing powder and a spot of salt.

- For sweet chaffles, you can include a tablespoon of keto-accommodating sugars like Confectioner's Swerve or Lakanto maple syrup. Remember Lily's chocolate chips!

INGREDIENTS
1 egg
1/2 cup cheddar, destroyed
1 tbsp almond flour (discretionary, see formula notes for different alternatives)

DIRECTIONS
1. Preheat the waffle creator as indicated by maker guidelines.

2. In a little blending bowl, combine egg and cheddar. Mix until all around consolidated.

3. Optionally, include the almond flour. See formula notes for more thoughts.

4. If utilizing a smaller than usual waffle producer, pour one portion of the waffle hitter into the waffle creator.

5. Cook for 3-4 minutes or until it arrives at wanted doneness. Rehash with the second 50% of the hitter.

NOTES

- See the formula varieties in the post above for thoughts regarding making lighter or fluffier waffles. You can make extremely scrumptious chaffles with simply the cheddar and egg.

- But, if you need lighter and fluffier chaffles, you can include either 1 teaspoonful of coconut flour and or 1 tablespoonful of the almond flour to the batter.

- You can likewise season your chaffle player with a spot of garlic powder, dried herbs, Italian flavouring, or everything Bagel flavouring.

- If you are utilizing a bigger size waffle producer, you might have the option to Cook the entire measure of hitter in one waffle. This will change with the size of your machine.

When beginning a keto diet, numerous individuals need to re-make their most loved non-keto foods to help with consistency on a keto diet. Numerous foods individuals look to re-make are bread, buns, biscuits, Cookies, brownies, cakes, tortillas, and numerous other flour-based foods.
In case you're fresh out of the plastic new to keto, below are a rundown of our preferred flours to use on a keto diet.

The best flours to to be taken on a keto diet

Coconut Flour is exceptionally high in fibre and low in carbohydrates, so it is immaculate to use in Prepared merchandise, for example, bread and desserts. Since it is high in fibre it typically just requires around 1/4 the sum if subbing instead of ordinary flour or the almond flour.

The Almond Flour is high in fat, and low in carbs, and moderate in protein. It is denser than coconut flour and is typically a 1:1 substitute for the standard flour, dissimilar to the coconut flour.

Psyllium Husk Flour is a flour that I had never utilized I begun to follow a ketogenic diet. It's high in fibre and is generally utilized in bread and move recipes.

Ground Flax Seed is high in fibre and fat and is pressed loaded with ALA Omega 3 fatties' acids.

Ground Chia Seeds are high in protein and fibre and have 0g net carbs per serving. They are extraordinary for utilizing in Prepared merchandise, yet I like utilizing ground chia for smoothies since it tends to not stick within the blender as customary chia seeds do.

Ground Sunflower Seeds. I've seen a great deal of pre-made Preparing blends utilize this as their flour of decision. They make for extremely chewy Cookies and brownies!

Cricket Flour. If you are feeling bold? Cricket flour has 2g fat, 1g carb and 7g protein per 10g serving.

Oat Fiber. With 3g of carbs all originating from fibre, this flour is flawless to add to Prepared great without the dread of spiking your glucose.

Wheat flour contains gluten—the protein that reinforces and ties mixture in Preparing. Along these lines, you will ordinarily need to source elective restricting specialists. Allude to what are the options to thickener or guar gum? For proposals.

In case you're following particular wheat-free or gluten-free formula it will have been deliberately detailed to get the ideal outcome utilizing the flour substitutes recorded. In the event that you are subbing other elective flours to those recorded you should know that you may get a disappointment, so don't do it just because you're cooking for a significant event.

A decent tip in the event that you do need to substitute a gluten-free flour is to utilize a flour of comparable properties and weight.

For instance, custard flour may substitute alright for arrowroot flour.

The flours recorded below are options in contrast to wheat, grain, or rye flours. Anyway, it is imperative to know that there is no accurate substitute for gluten-containing flour, and recipes made with wheat and gluten-free elective flours will be not quite the same as those containing wheat or gluten.

It's in every case better to store flours in hermetically sealed compartments in a dull, cool spot to maintain a strategic distance from them turning smelly. It's ideal to utilize them at room temperature; however, so measure out what you need and let them warm up somewhat.

Amaranth flour

Amaranth flour is produced using the seed of the Amaranth plant, which is a verdant vegetable. Amaranth seeds are high in protein, which makes a nutritious flour for Preparing—elective names: African spinach, Chinese spinach, Indian spinach, elephants ear.

Arrowroot flour

Arrowroot flour is ground from the foundation of the plant and is extremely valuable for thickening recipes. It is boring, and the fine powder turns out to be clear when it is cooked, which makes it perfect for clear thickening sauces.

Banana flour

It is produced using unripe green bananas that are dried and processed to make a flour that has a grain-like taste rather than a banana taste. Can be used for all Cooking and heating, or as a thickener for soups and sauces. Utilize 25% less banana flour than is proposed for flour in recipes.

Grain flour

The grain just contains a modest quantity of gluten, so is once in a while used to make bread, except for unleavened bread. It has a somewhat nutty flavour and can be utilized to thicken or enhance soups or stews. Mixed with other elective flours, it is additionally genuinely flexible for cakes, bread rolls, baked good, dumplings and so on.

Darker rice flour

Darker rice flour is heavier than its family member, white rice flour. It is processed from unpolished dark coloured rice, so it has a higher nutritional incentive than white, and as it contains the wheat of the darker rice, it has a higher fibre content. This additionally implies it has an observable surface, somewhat grainy.

It has a nutty taste, which sometimes turn out in recipes relying upon different ingredients, and the surface will likewise add to a heavier item than recipes made with white rice flour. It is a rare occurrence utilized totally all alone due to its heavier nature.

Mass purchasing isn't suggested as it is better utilized when crisp, store in an impenetrable compartment.

Buckwheat flour

Buckwheat flour isn't, regardless of its name a type of wheat, buckwheat is really identified with rhubarb. The little seeds of the plant are ground to make flour.

It has a solid nutty taste so isn't commonly utilized all alone in a formula, as the flavour of the completed item can be exceptionally overwhelming, and somewhat harsh—

elective names: beech wheat, kasha, Saracen corn.

Chia flour

Produced using ground chia seeds.Profoundly nutritious, chia seeds have been marked a "superfood" containing Omega 3, fibre, calcium and protein, all stuffed into little seeds.

Otherwise called "nature's rocket fuel" the same number of sportspeople and superathletes, for example, the Tarahumara use it for upgraded vitality levels during occasions.

On the off chance that chia flour isn't promptly accessible, at that point put chia seeds in a processor and whizz up a few. Whenever utilized in preparing, fluid levels and heating time may be expanded marginally.

Chickpea flour (otherwise called gram or garbanzo flour)

This is ground from chickpeas and has a solid marginally nutty taste. It isn't commonly utilized all alone.

Coconut flour

Produced using dried, defatted coconut meat this flour is high in fibre with a light coconut enhance. Commonly extra fluid will be required in a formula that utilizes coconut flour.

Coffee Flour

Produced using the disposed of espresso cherry natural product this is a nutritious flour that doesn't taste of espresso. The natural espresso product is processed into a flour that is high in fibre, and low in fat, which also has more iron than most grains, and is low in caffeine, and has more potassium than bananas.

Cornflour

Cornflour is processed from corn into a fine, white powder, and is utilized for thickening recipes and sauces. It has a dull taste, and in a this manner, is utilized related to different ingredients that will bestow flavour to the formula.

It additionally works very well when blended in with different flours, for instance, when making fine players for tempura.

A few sorts of cornflour are processed from wheat; however, are marked wheaten cornflour.

Cornmeal
Ground from corn. Heavier than cornflour, not for the most part compatible in recipes.

Hemp flour
Produced using ground hemp seeds it has a gentle, nutty flavour.

Lupin flour
Produced using a vegetable in a similar plant family as peanuts. It is increasingly high in protein and fibre, low in fat yet conveys a similar protein that causes hypersensitive responses/hypersensitivity to nut or vegetables, which makes it unsatisfactory for individuals with nut or vegetable sensitivities for example soybeans.

Maize flour
Ground from corn. Heavier than cornflour, not for the most part exchangeable in recipes.

Millet flour

Originates from the grass family, and is utilized as an oat in numerous African and Asian nations. It may be used to thicken soups and make level bread and frying pancakes. Since it comes up short on any type of gluten, it's not fit to numerous sorts of Preparing.

Oat flour

Ground from oats care should be taken to guarantee that it is sourced from a non-wheat tainting process. Likewise contains avenin, which is a protein like gluten, so even guaranteed gluten-free oats may not be appropriate for all celiacs.

Ingests fluids more than numerous flours, so may need to build the fluid substance of any formula it is added to. Promptly substitutes into many cakes and treat recipes. Oat flour goes foul rapidly, either purchase modest quantities or use rapidly, store it in the ice chest/cooler, or make your own utilizing a food processor.

Potato flour

This flour ought not to be mistaken for potato carbohydrate flour. Potato flour has a solid potato season and is a substantial flour, so a little goes far. Mass purchasing isn't suggested except if you are utilizing it all the time for an assortment of recipes as it doesn't have a long time span of usability.

Potato starch flour

This is a fine white flour produced using potatoes and has a light potato season which is imperceptible when utilized in recipes. It's one of only a handful, not many elective flours that keeps very much gave it is stored in a sealed shut container, and someplace cool and dim.

Quinoa flour

Quinoa is identified with the plant group of spinach and beets. It has been utilized for more than 5,000 years as a grain, and the Incas considered it the mother seed. Quinoa gives a decent wellspring of vegetable protein, and it is the seeds of the quinoa plant that are ground to make flour.

Rye flour

Rye flour is an emphatically seasoned flour, dull in shading. Bread made with rye flour is denser than those made with wheat, for instance, pumpernickel which is for all intents and purposes dark. Rye flour has a low gluten content, yet it can likewise be utilized for recipes, for example, hotcakes and biscuits.

Sorghum flour

Ground from sorghum grain, which is like millet. The flour is utilized to make porridge or level unleavened bread. It is a significant staple in Africa and India.
This flour stores well under typical temperatures.

Soya flour

Soya flour is a type of flour that is high protein flour with a nutty taste. It isn't commonly utilized all alone in recipes; however, when joined with different flours is fruitful as an elective flour. Can be utilized to thicken recipes or included as a flavour enhancer.
It should be painstakingly stored as it is a high-fat flour and can go rank if not stored appropriately. A cool, dim condition is prescribed and can even be stored in the fridge.

Custard flour

Custard flour is produced using the base of the cassava plant when ground it appears as a light, delicate, fine white flour. Custard flour adds chewiness to heating and is a decent thickener. Custard flour is a phenomenal expansion to any wheat-free kitchen. It's a genuinely strong flour, so putting away at room temperature is no issue.

Teff flour

Teff originates from the grass family and is a small oat grain local to northern Africa. It is currently finding a speciality in the health food advertising on the grounds that it is nutritious.

White rice flour

This flour is processed from cleaned white rice, so it is extremely dull in taste, and not especially nutritious. White rice flour is perfect for recipes that require a light surface; for instance, our herby dumplings. It very well may be utilized all alone for an assortment of recipes and has a sensible time span of usability, as long as it is stored in an impenetrable compartment to evade it retaining dampness from the air.

RECIPES FOR BASIC FLAVORED CHAFFLES

NUTTY SPREAD CUP CHAFFLES

Yield: 1 peanut butter cup chaffle

Prep time: 10 minutes

Cook time: 6 minutes

Total time: 16 minutes

Thick chocolate chaffles spread with a thick layer of smooth, sweet, nutty spread!

INGREDIENTS
For the chaffle:
1 huge egg
2 tablespoons cocoa powder
1 tablespoon sugar
1 tablespoon sugar freechocolate chips
1/4 teaspoon coffee powder

1/2 cup finely destroyed mozzarella

For the nutty spread filling:
3 tablespoons smooth nutty spread
2 tablespoons powdered sugar
1 tablespoon spread, mellowed

DIRECTIONS

To make the chaffles:
1. Plug in the waffle iron to preheat.

2. Whisk together the egg, cocoa powder, sugar, chocolate slashes, and coffee powder. Mix in the mozzarella.

3. Add a portion of the player to the waffle creator and Cook for 3 minutes. Rehash with outstanding player.

To make the nutty spread filling:
1. Add the entirety of the ingredients to a little bowl and mix together with a fork until smooth and velvety.

To amass:
1. Let waffles cool before spreading with the nutty spread and shutting to shape a sandwich.

NOTES

If you don't mind note that I've deducted sugar alcohols from this formula as erythritol, for the most part, has no impact on glucose. In the event that you include sugar alcohols in your carb check, you'll need to compute this yourself.

NUTRITION INFORMATION:

calories:210 | total fat: 15 | saturated fat: 5g | trans fat: 0g | unsaturated fat: 8g | cholesterol: 61mg | sodium: 208mg | carbohydrates: 4gnet | carbohydrates: 3g | fiber: 1g | sugar: 2g | protein: 8g.

LARGE MAC CHAFFLE

yield: 1 big mac

prep time: 10 minutes

cook time: 10 minutes

total time: 20 minutes

These cheeseburger chaffles pose a flavour like my preferred cheap food burger, directly down to the mystery ingredient! Don't hesitate to twofold or even fourfold this formula in case you're taking care of multiple!

INGREDIENTS

For the cheeseburgers:
1/3 pound ground hamburger
1/2 teaspoon garlic salt
 2 cuts American cheddar

For the Chaffles:
1 enormous egg
1/2 cup finely destroyed mozzarella
1/4 teaspoon garlic salt

For the Big Mac Sauce:
2 teaspoons mayonnaise
1 teaspoon ketchup
1 teaspoon dill pickle relish
 splash vinegar, to taste

To collect:
2 tablespoons destroyed lettuce
3-4 dill pickles
 2 teaspoons minced onion

DIRECTIONS
To make the burgers:
1. Warm an iron over medium-high warmth.

2. Partition the ground hamburger into 2
equivalent measured balls and spot each on
the frying pan, at any rate, 6 inches
separated.

3. Let Cook for 1 moment.

4. Utilize a little serving of mixed greens
plate to immovably squeeze straight down
on the bundles of hamburger to straighten.
Sprinkle with garlic salt.

5. Cook 2 minutes or until mostly cooked through. Flip the burgers cautiously and sprinkle with outstanding garlic salt.

6. Keep cooking 2 minutes or until cooked through.

7. Spot one cut of cheddar over every patty and afterwards stack the patties and put aside on a plate. Spread with foil.

To make the chaffles:
1. Warmth the smaller than normal waffle iron and splash with non-stick shower.

2. Whisk together the egg, cheddar, and garlic salt until very much consolidated.

3. Include half of the egg blend to the waffle iron and Cook for 2-3 minutes. Put in a safe spot and rehash with an outstanding player.

To make the Big Mac Sauce:
1. Whisk together all ingredients.

To amass burgers:
1. Top one chaffle with the stacked burger patties, destroyed lettuce, pickles, and onions.

2. Spread the Big Mac sauce over the other chaffle and spot sauce side down over the sandwich.

3. Eat right away.

NOTES
Don't hesitate to twofold or fourfold this formula.

NUTRITION INFORMATION:

calories: 831 | total fat: 56g | saturated fat: 23g | trans fat: 2g | unsaturated fat: 26g | cholesterol: 382mg | sodium: 3494mg | carbohydrates: 8g | net carbohydrates: 6g | fiber: 2g | sugar: 2g | protein: 65g

GARLIC BREAD CHAFFLE

yield: 2 servings

prep time: 5 minutes

cook time: 10 minutes

total time: 15 minutes

Gooey garlic bread made in minutes on account of your waffle producer!

INGREDIENTS
1 huge egg
1/2 cup finely destroyed mozzarella
1 teaspoon coconut flour
¼ teaspoon Preparing powder
½ teaspoon garlic powder
1 tablespoon spread, softened
1/4 teaspoon garlic salt
2 tablespoons Parmesan
1 teaspoon minced parsley

DIRECTIONS

1. Plug in your small waffle iron to preheat. Preheat broiler to 375 degrees.

2. Add the egg, mozzarella, coconut flour, Preparing powder, and garlic powder to a blending bowl and whisk well to join.

3. Pour a portion of the chaffle hitter into the waffle iron and Cook for 3 minutes or until the steam stops. Spot the chaffle on a heating sheet.

4. Repeat with the remaining chaffle hitter.

5. Stir together the margarine and garlic salt and brush over the chaffles.

6. Top the chaffles with the Parmesan.

7. Place the container in the broiler for 5 minutes to liquefy the cheddar.

8. Sprinkle with parsley before serving.

NOTES

The garlic salt makes these somewhat salty -
don't hesitate to swap in crisp minced garlic
or garlic powder, in case you're watching
salt.

NUTRITION INFORMATION:

calories: 186 | total fat: 14g | saturated fat:
8g | trans fat: 0g | unsaturated fat: 5g |
cholesterol: 127mg | sodium: 590mg |
carbohydrates: 3g | net carbohydrates: 2g |
fiber: 1g | sugar: 1g | protein: 10g

BASIC CHAFFLE RECIPE

Yield: 2 waffles

Prep time: 1 minute

Cook time: 6 minutes

Total time: 7 minutes

These chaffles are only two ingredients and Cook in only a couple of moments! Flawless spread with margarine and sugar-free syrup.

INGREDIENTS
1 enormous egg
1/2 cup finely destroyed mozzarella

DIRECTIONS
1. Plugin the waffle producer to warm.

2. Break the egg into a little bowl and race with a fork. Add the mozzarella and mix to consolidate.

3. Spray the waffle iron with non-stick shower.

4. Pour a portion of the egg blend into the warmed waffle iron and cook for 2-3 minutes.

5. Remove waffle cautiously and cook remaining player.

6. Serve warm with margarine and without sugar syrup.

NOTES
Have a go at including a sprinkle of vanilla or run of cinnamon for next-level breakfast chaffles!

NUTRITION INFORMATION:
calories: 202 | total fat: 13g | saturated fat: 6g | trans fat: 0g| unsaturated fat: 5g| cholesterol: 214mg| sodium: 364mg| carbohydrates: 3g | net carbohydrates: 3g| fiber: 0g | sugar: 1g | protein: 16g

STRAWBERRY SHORTCAKE CHAFFLE

Prep Time: 4 minutes

Cook Time: 12 minutes

Servings: 3 Chaffles

This low carb and keto benevolent Strawberry Shortcake Chaffle is the ideal dessert to appreciate after dinner!

INGREDIENTS
Strawberry besting Ingredients
3 new strawberries
1/2 tablespoon granulated swerve

Sweet Chaffle Ingredients
1 tablespoon almond flour
1/2 cup mozzarella cheddar
1 egg
1 tablespoon granulated swerve
1/4 teaspoon vanilla concentrate
Keto Whipped Cream

DIRECTIONS

1. Heat up your waffle creator. If you are utilizing a smaller than usual waffle producer this formula will make 2 chaffles, if utilizing a huge waffle creator, this formula will make 1 enormous sweet chaffle.

2. Rinse and slash up your new strawberries. Spot the strawberries in a little bowl and include 1/2 tablespoon granulated swerve. Blend the strawberries in with the swerve and put in a safe spot.

3. In a bowl blend the almond flour, egg, mozzarella cheddar, granulated swerve and vanilla concentrate.

4. Pour 1/3 of the player into your smaller than usual waffle creator and cook for 3-4 minutes. At that point cook another 1/3 of the player and the remainder of the hitter to make 3 keto chaffles.

5. While your second chaffle is cooking, make your keto whipped cream in the event that you don't have any available.

6. Assemble your Strawberry Shortcake Chaffle by putting whipped cream and strawberries on your sweet chaffle. At that point sprinkle the juice that will likewise be in the bowl with the strawberries on top.

NUTRITION INFORMATION
Calories: 112kcal | Carbohydrates: 2g| Protein: 7g | Fat: 8g | Saturated Fat: 3g | Cholesterol: 69mg | Sodium: 138mg | Potassium: 53mg | Fiber: 1g | Sugar: 1g | Vitamin A: 205IU | Vitamin C: 7mg | Calcium: 107mg | Iron: 1mg

KETO BLUEBERRY CHAFFLE

This delectable keto blueberry waffle is in fact called a Keto Chaffle! Furthermore, a kid is it delish! Consummately sweet, with succulent blueberries, these blueberry keto chaffles taste extraordinary and are low carb and keto agreeable.

Prep Time: 3 minutes

Cook Time: 15 minutes

Servings: 5 Chaffles

INGREDIENTS
1 cup of mozzarella cheddar
2 tablespoons almond flour
1 tsp heating powder
2 eggs
1 tsp cinnamon
2 tsp of Swerve
3 tablespoon blueberries

DIRECTIONS

1. Heat up your Dash smaller than expected waffle producer.

2. In a blending, bowl include the mozzarella cheddar, almond flour, heating powder, eggs, cinnamon, swerve and blueberries. Blend well, so all the ingredients are combined.

3. Spray your smaller than expected waffle producer with non-stick Cooking shower.

4. Add shortly under 1/4 a cup of blueberry keto waffle player.

5. Close the top and cook the chaffle for 3-5 minutes. Check it at the 3-minute imprint to check whether it is fresh and darker. In the event that it isn't or it adheres to the highest point of the waffle machine close the cover and cook for 1-2 minutes longer.

6. Serve with a sprinkle of swerving confectioners' sugar or keto syrup.

NUTRITIONAL INFORMATION

Calories: 115kcal | Carbohydrates: 5g | Protein: 8g | Fat: 8.5g | Saturated Fat: 4g |

Cholesterol: 84mg | Sodium: 165mg | Potassium: 142mg | Fiber: 1g | Sugar: 1g | Vitamin A: 245IU | Vitamin C: 1mg | Calcium: 178mg | Iron: 1mg

KETO CHAFFLE GARLIC CHEESY BREAD STICKS

Prep Time: 3 minutes

Cook Time: 7 minutes

Total Time: 10 minutes

Servings: 8 sticks

INGREDIENTS
1 medium egg
1/2 cup mozzarella cheddar ground
2 tablespoons almond flour
1/2 teaspoon garlic powder
1/2 teaspoon oregano
1/2 teaspoon salt

Besting
2 tablespoons spread, unsalted mellowed
1/2 teaspoon garlic powder
1/4 cup mozzarella cheddar ground

DIRECTIONS
1. Turn on your waffle creator and daintily oil it (I give it a light shower with olive oil)

2. In a bowl, beat the egg.

3. Add the mozzarella, almond flour, garlic powder, oregano and salt and blend well.

4. Spoon the hitter into your waffle creator (mine is a square twofold waffle, and this blend covers both waffle areas. In the event that you are utilizing a littler waffle creator spoon a large portion of the blend in at once).

5. I spoon my blend into the focal point of my waffle creator and tenderly spread it out towards the edges.

6. Close the cover of the pot and cook for 5 minutes.

7. Using tongs, expel the cooked waffles and cut into 4 strips for each waffle.

8. Place the sticks on a plate and pre-heat the flame broil.

9. Mix the margarine with the garlic powder and spread over the sticks.

10. Sprinkle the mozzarella over the sticks and spot under the flame broil for 2-3 minutes until the cheddar has dissolved and percolating.

11. Eat right away! (If we have gobbled this warmed up yet are a lot more pleasant crisply made)

NOTES

The net carbohydrates will then be the Total carb check less the fiber tally. Carb tally prohibits sugar alcohols.

Varieties may happen for different reasons, including item accessibility and food

Preparation. We make no portrayal or guarantee of the precision of this data.

NUTRITION INFORMATION
Calories: 74kcal | Carbohydrates: 0.9g | Protein: 3.4g | Fat: 6.5g | Fiber: 0.2g

KETO SALTED CARAMEL FRAPPUCCINO

In the event that you are needing your ordinary frappuccino from Starbucks and are keto/Low Carb, at that point you are going to cherish this Keto Salted Caramel Frappuccino!

Prep Time: 5 minutes

Cook Time: 5 minutes

Total Time: 10 minutes

Servings: 1

INGREDIENTS

1 mug espresso solidified in an ice plate
1 mug espresso
3 tablespoons overwhelming cream
3 tablespoons without sugar caramel syrup
5 drops fluid stevia extricate
tablespoon without sugar caramel sauce
sprinkle

DIRECTIONS

1. In the blender, add the espresso ice 3D squares, espresso, substantial cream, caramel syrup, and stevia.

2. Blend it for 30 seconds, or until smooth.

3. While the drink is mixing, get your premade got cream or whip ready a bunch of keto whipped cream.

4. Place the whipped cream in a cake pack with a star tip.

5. Take your cup and include a twirl of the caramel around within the cup.

6. Pour the Frappuccino blend into the cup and top it with the whipped cream.

NUTRITION INFORMATION

Calories: 159kcal | Carbohydrates: 2g | Protein: 1g | Fat: 16g | Saturated Fat: 10g | Cholesterol: 61mg | Sodium: 26mg | Potassium: 232mg | Vitamin A: 660IU | Calcium: 29mg

CATCHPHRASES KETO SALTED CARAMEL FRAPPUCCINO

The Keto Cheese Chips made in the Microwave are a delectable and fast Keto nibble. They are likewise ideal for including top of servings of mixed greens!

Prep Time: 1 minute

Cook Time: 1 minute

Total Time: 2 minutes

Servings:1

INGREDIENTS
3 ounces Sharp Cheddar Cheese Roughly
6 cuts of full-sized cheddar cuts

DIRECTIONS
1. Line a microwave-safe plate with a bit of material paper.

2. If you are utilizing full-size bits of cheddar, cut your cheddar cut into fourths. If you are using a square of cheddar you have to cut your cheddar here, and in the event that you are utilizing pre-cut cheddar, you can skirt this progression.

3. Arrange the cheddar on the plate, making a point to leave room between the cuts, so they don't run together.

4. Microwave on high for one moment.

5. Remove the material paper from the plate and allow the cheddar to cool.

6. If any of the chips liquefied together, you can cautiously break them separated or simply appreciate a huge chip.

NOTES

Nutrition data is dependent on 3 ounces of Sharp Cheddar Cheese, anyway, most cheddar has 0 carbs, so regardless of what cheddar you are utilizing you will at present have a 0 carb cheddar chip.

NUTRITION INFORMATION

Calories: 342kcal | Protein: 21g | Fat: 28g | Saturated Fat: 17g | Cholesterol: 89mg | Sodium: 528mg | Potassium: 83mg | Vitamin A: 850IU | Calcium: 613mg | Iron: 0.6mg

GREEK MARINATED FETA AND OLIVES

A heavenly Mediterranean diet propelled starter or bite, that is likewise low carb, these marinated olives and feta cheddar are ideal for any individual who is searching for an easy delectable formula.

Prep Time: 5 minutes

Cook Time: 5 minutes

Cool: 15 minutes

Servings: 4

INGREDIENTS
1 cup olive oil
1/4 teaspoon oregano
1/4 teaspoon thyme

1/2 teaspoon dried rosemary
1 cup kalamata olives
1 cup of green olives
1/2 pound feta

DIRECTIONS
1. In a little pan heat the oil, oregano, thyme, rosemary together over medium warmth for 5 minutes to inject the oil with the herbs.

2. Set the oil to the side and allow it to cool for 15 minutes.

3. Cut the feta into 1/2 inch shapes.

4. In a medium combining bowl tenderly mix the oil, olives, and feta.

5. Transfer into a sealed shut compartment, and store in the ice chest. You need the olives to marinate for at any rate 20 minutes before you eat them.

6. Serve the olives at room temperature. You should take the olives out a tad before serving them, so the olive oils heat up.

NUTRITION INFORMATION
Calories: 296kcal | Carbohydrates: 5g | Protein: 9g | Fat: 28g | Saturated Fat: 11g | Cholesterol: 50mg | Sodium: 1683mg | Potassium: 64mg | Fiber: 2g | Sugar: 3g | Vitamin A: 505IU | Calcium: 315mg | Iron: 0.7mg

CAPRESE SKEWERS

Prep Time: 14 minutes

Marinating Time: 3 hours

Total Time: 3 hours 14 minutes

Servings: 14 sticks

INGREDIENTS
14 Mozzarella balls Bocconcini
14 cherry tomatoes
14 basil leaves
7 dark olives cut down the middle

marinade
3 tablespoons olive oil
1 garlic clove hacked

1 teaspoon oregano dried
1/2 teaspoon salt
1/2 teaspoon dark pepper

DIRECTIONS
1. Mix the marinade in a Ziplock sack (or bowl with cover)

2. Add the tomato and bocconcini (mozzarella balls). Shake well and marinate for at least 3 hours (medium-term is perfect).

3. Assemble the tomatoes, cheddar on a medium estimated toothpick. Include a large portion of olive the top with a leaf of basil.

4. Drizzle any outstanding marinade or pesto to serve.

NOTES
Varieties may happen for different reasons, including item accessibility and food Preparation. We make no portrayal or guarantee of the precision of this data.

NUTRITION INFORMATION

Calories: 64kcal | Carbohydrates: 1.1g | Protein: 2.7g | Fat: 5.6g | Fiber: 0.3g

CAULIFLOWER CHEESE JALAPENO SOUP

Prep Time: 10 minutes

Cook Time: 40 minutes

Total Time: 50 minutes

Servings: 6 servings

INGREDIENTS

1 head cauliflower cut into florets
2 tablespoons olive oil
1 medium onion stripped and hacked
3 cloves garlic stripped and hacked
4 jalapeno peppers deseeded and hacked
500 ml stock - either vegetable or chicken
2 cups cheddar ground

1 teaspoon salt
1 teaspoon dark pepper

DIRECTIONS

1. Heat the olive oil in a huge pan on a medium warmth and include the cauliflower florets. Cook for around 5-8 minutes, turning much of the time until marginally brilliant in shading.

2. Add the onion, the garlic and the jalapeno and then cook for a further 3 minutes.

3. Add stock and bring to the bubble, spread, and stew for around 20 minutes until the cauliflower is delicate.

4. Add the cheddar and season to taste. Cook for around 5 minutes until the cheddar has softened.

5. Remove from the warmth and mix either by utilizing a hand blender or emptying the soup into a blender.

6. Serve, gulp and appreciate!

NOTES

Other ground cheddar can be utilized. Attempt a Gruyere.

The Total carbs will now be the Total carb tally less the fibre tally. Carb tally prohibits sugar alcohols.

Varieties may happen for different reasons, including item accessibility and food Preparation. We make no portrayal or guarantee of the exactness of this data.

NUTRITION INFORMATION

Calories: 180kcal | Carbohydrates: 6.2g | Protein: 11g | Fat: 13g | Fiber: 2.1g

MUSHROOM TARRAGON SOUP

Prep Time: 5 minutes

Cook Time: 30 minutes

Servings: 4 servings

INGREDIENTS
8 oz white mushrooms slashed
1 onion, medium stripped and slashed
3 garlic cloves stripped and hacked
1 oz spread
2 tablespoon new tarragon hacked
2 cups vegetable or chicken stock
1 oz mascarpone cheddar
1 teaspoon salt
1 teaspoon dark pepper

DIRECTIONS

1. In a pot heat the spread on a medium warmth

2. Cook the onion and the garlic for 5 min.

3. Add the mushrooms and tenderly cook for 5 minutes. Spread with a cover to ensured the mushroom juices turn out.

4. Season with the salt and pepper.

5. Add the stock and mix well.

6. Add the new tarragon and stew for 15 minutes.

7. Stir in the mascarpone cheddar.

8. Either fill in as stout or fill a blender and mix for a smooth soup.

NOTES

Mascarpone can be subbed with overwhelming cream or coconut cream.

The net carbs will be the Total carb check less the fibre tally. Carb check prohibits sugar alcohols.

Varieties may happen for different reasons, including item accessibility and food Preparation. We make no portrayal or guarantee of the precision of this data.

NUTRITION INFORMATION

Calories: 121kcal | Carbohydrates: 7.4g | Protein: 3.1g | Fat: 9.3g | Fiber: 1.9g

KETO CHAFFLE BREAKFAST AND BRUNCH RECIPES

KETO COCONUT FLOUR WAFFLES RECIPE

This easy coconut flour waffles formula takes only 5 minutes to Prep + 5 minutes to Cook! Keto waffles with coconut flour make a delectable, without nut low carb breakfast.

Course: Breakfast

Cooking: American

Calories: 474 kcal

Prep Time: 5 minutes

Cook Time: 5 minutes

Total Time: 10 minutes

INGREDIENTS

3 tbsp Coconut flour

3 huge Eggs

2 oz Cream cheddar

2 tbsp of butter (or coconut oil)

1/4 cup of the Heavy cream (or any milk you like)

1 tbsp Erythritol (or any sugar)

1/2 tsp sans gluten heating powder

1/4 tsp Xanthan gum (discretionary, however, helps keep it together better)

1/2 tsp Vanilla concentrate (discretionary)

DIRECTIONS

1. Preheat your waffle creator.

2. Combine all ingredients in a blender. Puree until smooth.

3. Let the hitter sit for a couple of moments to thicken. It ought to be thicker than a pourable hitter, however easy to spread. In the event that it's brittle like treat mixture, include more milk or cream, a tablespoon at once, until it's increasingly similar to a thick hitter.

4. Scoop a meagre 1 cup (128 grams) player into the waffle producer, spread and spread. Cook, as indicated by producer guidelines (for the most part around 4-5 minutes), or until steam, is never again turning out the sides. Cautiously expel the waffle from the iron (it's delicate while it's hot).

5. Repeat with the residual hitter.

6. Optional advance: For crisper waffles, heat them in the broiler on a stove safe cooling rack for two or three minutes at 400 degrees F (204 degrees C), or in a toaster broiler.

NUTRITION INFORMATION
Calories | Fat41g | Protein14g | Total Carbs10g | Net Carbs7g | Fiber3g | Sugar3g

MOMENT POT SOUS VIDE EGG BITES RECIPE

This 4-fixing, easy Instant Pot sous vide egg nibbles formula is much the same as Starbucks! Perceive how to make sous vide egg chomps in the Instant Pot, including bacon gruyere and different flavours.

Course: Breakfast

Food: French

Calories: 227 kcal

Prep Time: 10 minutes

Cook Time: 9 minutes

Total Time: 19 minutes

Serving size: 1 egg chomp

INGREDIENTS
5 enormous Eggs
1/2 cup Gruyere cheddar (destroyed)
1/3 cup Heavy cream
2 tbsp Water (in addition to 1 cup more to fill the Instant Pot)
1/8 tsp Sea salt
1/8 tsp Black pepper
7 cuts Bacon (Cooked)

DIRECTIONS
1. Grease a silicone egg nibble form with margarine or olive oil.

2. Stack the bacon cuts and cut them down the middle. Spot 2 bits of bacon next to each other into the base of the form, bending up the sides.

3. Blend the eggs, cheddar, cream, 2 tablespoons (29 ml) water, ocean salt, and dark pepper in a blender at rapid, until smooth and somewhat foamy. (Then again, you can utilize a hand blender in a bowl.)

4. Pour the egg blend equally into the moulds. Spread the shaping plate firmly with foil.

5. Pour 1 cup approximately (236 ml) of water into the Instant Pot and spot the trivet with handles inside. Cautiously place the egg chomp shape onto the trivet. Close the cover, set the steam valve to Seal, press the Manual catch, and set the time to 9 minutes at High weight.

6. When time is up, sit tight for 5 minutes of normal steam discharge.

7. Use broiler gloves to lift the trivet out of the weight Cooker. Evacuate the thwart and allow them to cool for 5 minutes (they will contract), at that point flip the form over a plate and jump out.

NUTRITION INFORMATION
Calories227 | Fat20g | Protein11g | Total Carbs1g | Net Carbs0g | Fiber1g | Sugar1g

THE LOW CARB PALEO KETO BLUEBERRY AND THE MUFFINS RECIPE WITH ALMOND FLOUR

Perceive how to make the best keto biscuits in only 30 minutes! These ultra sodden almond flour blueberry biscuits without any Preparation are brisk and easy. It's the ideal low carb paleo blueberry biscuits formula - and the just a single you'll ever require.

Course: Breakfast, Snack

Cooking: American

Calories: 217 kcal

Prep Time: 10 minutes

Cook Time: 20 minutes

Total Time: 30 minutes

Serving size: 1 biscuit

INGREDIENTS

2 1/2 cup Blanched almond flour

1/2 cup Erythritol (or any granulated sugar)

1 1/2 tsp without gluten heating powder

1/4 tsp Sea salt (discretionary, yet prescribed)

1/3 cup Coconut oil (estimated strong, at that point liquefied; can likewise utilize margarine)

1/3 cup Unsweetened almond milk

3 huge Eggs

1/2 tsp Vanilla concentrate

3/4 cup Blueberries

DIRECTIONS

1. Pre-heat the stove to 350 degrees F (177 degrees C). Line a biscuit skillet with 10 or 12 silicone or material paper biscuit liners. (Utilize 12 for lower calories/carbs, or 10 for bigger biscuit tops.)

2. In an enormous bowl, mix together the almond flour, erythritol, Preparing powder and ocean salt.

3. Mix in the softened coconut oil, almond milk, eggs, and vanilla concentrate—crease in the blueberries.

4. Distribute the hitter equally among the biscuit cups. Heat for around 20-25 minutes, until the top is brilliant and an embedded toothpick tells the truth.

NUTRITION INFORMATION
Calories217 | Fat19g | Protein7g | Total Carbs6g | Net Carbs3g | Fiber3g | Sugar2g

KETO MATCHA GREEN TEA FRAPPE RECIPE

Perceive how to make a matcha green tea frappe at home with only 5 ingredients + 5 minutes! My easy keto green tea frappe formula is without sugar, yet tastes simply like the bistro ones.

Course: Breakfast, Drinks

Food: American

Calories: 156 kcal

Cook Time: 5 minutes

Total Time: 5 minutes

INGREDIENTS
3/4 cup of unsweetened almond milk (or coconut milk for sans nut)
2 tbsp of heavy cream
1/2 tbsp of Zulay Kitchen Matcha Green Tea
1 cup of Ice
 1 tbsp Powdered erythritol (or any fluid or powdered sugar, discretionary)

1/2 tsp Vanilla concentrate (discretionary)
Whipped cream (discretionary, for fixing - utilize natively constructed without sugar)

DIRECTIONS

1. Combine everything with the exception of whipped cream in a blender. Mix until wanted consistency is come to.

2. If wanted, modify sugar or matcha to taste.

3. Pour into a glass or container. Top with whipped cream.

NUTRITION INFORMATION

Calories156 | Fat13g | Protein5g | Total Carbs2g | Net Carbs2g | Fiber0g | Sugar1g

KETO PUMPKIN SPICE LATTE RECIPE

My mystery stunt for how to make a healthy pumpkin flavour latte at home, in only 5 minutes! This healthy keto pumpkin zest latte formula suggests a flavour like one from a café, without the sugar. You'll never figure this is a low carb without sugar pumpkin flavour latte.

Course: Breakfast, Snack

Food: American

Calories: 144 kcal

Prep Time: 2 minutes

Cook Time: 3 minutes

Total Time: 5 minutes

Serving size: 1 pumpkin flavour latte

INGREDIENTS

3/4 cup of almond milk

2 tbsp of Heavy cream

2 tbsp pumpkin puree

2 tsp Xylitol (or other sugar of decision, to taste)

1/4 tsp Pumpkin pie zest (in addition to additional for sprinkling)

1/4 tsp Vanilla concentrate

1/2 cup Brewed solid espresso (or 1/4 mug coffee)

Whipped cream (for serving)

DIRECTIONS

1. Microwave technique: Stir together the almond milk, substantial cream, pumpkin puree, xylitol, and pumpkin pie zest in a 12-ounce mug. Microwave it for about 45 to 60 seconds, until hot.

Stove-top technique: Stir together the almond milk, substantial cream, pumpkin puree, xylitol, and pumpkin pie zest in a little pot, until hot. Fill a 12-ounce mug.

2. Add the vanilla concentrate. Utilize a milk frother to mix until the blend is smooth and foamy, and sugar has disintegrated.

3. Stir in the blended espresso. Top it up with the whipped cream and a sprinkle of pumpkin pie zest (discretionary).

NUTRITION INFORMATION
Calories144 | Fat13g | Protein2g | Total Carbs4g | Net Carbs3g | Fiber1g | Sugar2g

HEALTHY KETO ZUCCHINI PANCAKES RECIPE

Perceive how to make a healthy zucchini flapjacks formula in only 20 minutes, with 6 ingredients! Keto squash hotcakes are fleecy, flavorful, and delightful.

Course: Breakfast, Main Course

Food: Russian

Calories: 204 kcal

Prep Time: 10 minutes

Cook Time: 10 minutes

Total Time: 20 minutes

Serving size: 3 enormous flapjacks

INGREDIENTS

3 cups Yellow squash or zucchini (ground)
1 tsp Sea salt (isolated)
3 enormous Egg
1/2 cup Full-fat buttermilk (or full-fat kefir)
3/4 cup Blanched almond flour

1/2 tsp Baking pop

Olive oil (or any oil of decision for singing)

DIRECTIONS

1. Set the ground squash in a colander over the sink and sprinkle with 1/2 teaspoon ocean salt. Let it sit for in any event 10 minutes.

2. Wrap the zucchini into a kitchen towel and bend over the sink to wring out any additional water. Attempt to discharge however much as could reasonably be expected, until the remaining ground zucchini is dry and not watery.

3. In a huge bowl, consolidate the almond flour, Preparing pop, and staying 1/2 teaspoon ocean salt. Beat in the eggs. Mix in buttermilk and squash.

4. Pour inadequate 1/4-cup-size (60 mL) circles of the hitter onto the container. Spread and cook for 2-3 minutes, until the base is brilliant and edges are dry. Flip and rehash on the opposite side.

NUTRITION INFORMATION
Calories204 | Fat15g | Protein10g | Total Carbs8g | Net Carbs5g | Fiber3g | Sugar4g

LOW CARB CHOCOLATE PROTEIN PANCAKES RECIPE

Figure out how to make protein hotcakes! This low carb chocolate protein flapjacks formula (protein powder hotcakes) takes only 20 minutes and has 11g protein per serving.

Course: Breakfast

Food: American

Calories: 237 kcal

Prep Time: 10 minutes

Cook Time: 10 minutes

Total Time: 20 minutes

INGREDIENTS

1/2 cup of Whey protein powder (or collagen, or egg white protein powder)

1/2 cup of blanched almond flour

3 tbsp of cocoa powder

3 tbsp of erythritol (or sugar of decision)

1 tsp sans of gluten preparing powder

4 big eggs

1/3 cup of almond milk

2 tbsp of avocado oil (or liquefied coconut oil)

1 tsp of vanilla concentrate

1/8 tsp of sea salt

DIRECTIONS

1. Shake all the ingredients together in the Whiskware Batter Mixer. Let the player sit for 5 minutes.

2. Preheat a dish over medium-low warmth. Crush player into the container to shape little circles (3 crawls in width). Spread with a top and cook for two or three minutes, until bubbles structure on top. Utilize an exceptionally slim turner to deliberately flip the hotcakes, at that point cook for two or three minutes on the opposite side.

3. Repeat with the rest of the player.

NUTRITION INFORMATION
Calories237 | Fat20g | Protein11g | Total Carbs7g | Net Carbs5g | Fiber2g | Sugar0g

EASY VANILLA LOW CARB PROTEIN WAFFLES RECIPE

How to make protein waffles? EASY! This low carb high protein waffles formula (protein powder waffles) is only 5 ingredients and Prepared in under 10 minutes!

Course: Breakfast

Food: American

Calories: 439 kcal

Prep Time: 2 minutes

Cook Time: 5 minutes

Total Time: 7 minutes

Serving size: 1/2 enormous Belgian waffle

INGREDIENTS
2 scoops Atkins Vanilla Protein Powder (1/4 cup)
2 tbsp Peanut margarine (smooth, no sugar included)
2 tbsp Coconut oil (softened)
3 enormous Eggs
1/2 tsp sans gluten Preparing powder
1/4 tsp Sea salt

DIRECTIONS
1. Incoporate the ingredients into a blender, and mix until smooth.

2. Preheat your waffle iron. Move the player into the waffle iron (it will be thick) and appropriate equally.

3. Cook as indicated by producer's directions. Regularly the waffle cooks for 4-5 minutes, and is done when steam is never again turning out.

NUTRITION INFORMATION

Calories439 | Fat32g | Protein29g | Total Carbs11g | Net Carbs5g | Fiber6g | Sugar2g

IMMACULATE BAKED HARD BOILED EGGS IN THE OVEN

cooking eggs in the stove is easy! Prepare hard bubbled eggs in the broiler take 20-30 minutes. for both delicate or hard bubbled eggs, here's a time chart for how to bubble eggs in the stove.

Course: Breakfast

Cooking: American

Calories: 70 kcal

Cook Time: 30 minutes

Total Time: 30 minutes

Servings: 12 eggs

INGREDIENTS
12 huge Eggs

DIRECTIONS

1. Preheat the stove to 325 degrees F (163 degrees C).

2. Place 1 egg in every cup in a biscuit tin.

3. Bake the eggs for 20 to 30 min. for your ideal degree of doneness. Eggs in the stove will take 20 minutes for delicate bubbled, 30 minutes for completely hard bubbled. See the diagram in the post above for Preparing times in the middle.

4. Meanwhile, prepare a pot of ice water. When you expel the eggs from the broiler.

NUTRITION INFORMATION
Calories70 | Fat5g | Protein7g | Total Carbs0g | Net Carbs0g | Fiber0g | Sugar0g

EASY LOW CARB-KETO OATMEAL RECIPE

Figure out how to make keto oatmeal 4 different ways - maple walnut, strawberries and cream, chocolate nutty spread, or cinnamon roll - all dependent on an easy low carb oatmeal formula with 5 ingredients!

Course: Breakfast

Cooking: American

Calories: 592 kcal

Prep Time: 5 minutes

Cook Time: 3 minutes

Total Time: 8 minutes

INGREDIENTS
Basic Keto Oatmeal
1/4 cup hemp seeds (hulled hemp seeds)
1 tbsp golden flaxseed meal
1 tbsp vital proteins collagen peptides

1/2 tbsp chia seeds

1/2 cup of coconut milk (from a bowl; 1/2 fluid and 1/2 thick cream; or simply overwhelming cream if not without dairy)

Discretionary Add-Ins (Recommended for all varieties)

1 tbsp erythritol (to taste)

1 squeeze sea salt (to taste)

Maple Pecan Add-Ins

1/2 tsp Maple extricate

2 tbsp Pecans (hacked)

Chocolate Peanut Butter

1 tbsp peanut spread

1 tbsp coconut milk (or almond milk)

1 tbsp without sugar dull chocolate chips

Strawberries and Cream Add-Ins

2 tbsp strawberries (finely hacked)

1/2 tsp Vanilla concentrate

2 tbsp Coconut cream (or simply the cream part from canned coconut milk, or overwhelming cream if not without dairy)

Cinnamon Roll Add-Ins

3/4 tsp cinnamon

3/4 tsp vanilla concentrate (separated into 1/2 tsp and 1/4 tsp)

1 tbsp Powdered erythritol

1/2 tbsp Coconut cream (or simply the cream part from canned coconut milk, or overwhelming cream if not without dairy)

DIRECTIONS
Basic Keto Oatmeal
1. Stir all ingredients, with the exception of cream or milk, together in a little pot. (This incorporates the discretionary sugar and salt if utilizing.)

2. Add cream/milk and speed until smooth.

Stovetop directions:
Stew for a couple of moments, until thickened.

Microwave directions:
Rather than a pan, utilize a microwave-safe bowl. Warmth for 1 to 2 minutes, until thickened.

Serve quickly, or follow choices below for include ins.

Maple Pecan Keto Oatmeal
1. Stir in the maple extricate and cleaved walnuts.

Chocolate Peanut Butter Keto Oatmeal

1. Stir in the nutty spread and additional milk, at that point stew for one more moment.

2. Stir in chocolate chips.

Strawberries and Cream Keto Oatmeal

1. Stir in strawberries, coconut cream, and vanilla concentrate.

Cinnamon Roll Keto Oatmeal

1. Stir in cinnamon and 1/2 tsp (2.5 mL) vanilla concentrate.

2. In an extremely little bowl, whisk together powdered sugar, coconut cream, and 1/4 tsp (1.25 mL) vanilla concentrate—shower over oatmeal in a twirling design.

NUTRITION INFORMATION
Calories592 | Fat47g | Protein31g | Total Carbs9g | Net Carbs4g | Fiber5g | Sugar1g

LOW CARB DOUBLE CHOCOLATE PROTEIN MUFFINS RECIPE

These low carb twofold chocolate protein biscuits are easy to make, damp and heavenly. This healthy protein biscuit formula needs only 10 minutes Prep time!

Course: Breakfast, Dessert

Cooking: American

Calories: 233 kcal

Prep Time: 10 minutes

Cook Time: 25 minutes

Total Time: 35 minutes

Serving size: 1 biscuit

INGREDIENTS
2 cup blanched almond flour
2/3 cup allulose (or any granulated sugar)
1/2 cup Cocoa powder
1/4 cup vital proteins collagen peptides
1 1/2 tsp sans gluten heating powder

1/4 tsp sea salt

1/3 cup coconut oil

1/2 cup unsweetened almond milk

3 enormous eggs

1/2 tsp vanilla concentrate

3/4 cup sans sugar dim chocolate chips

DIRECTIONS

1. Preheat the broiler to 350 degrees F (177 degrees C). Line a biscuit container with 12 material paper liners or silicone biscuit liners.

2. In an enormous bowl, mix together the almond flour, sugar, cocoa powder, collagen peptides, Preparing powder and ocean salt.

3. Stir in the liquefied coconut oil and almond milk. Rush in the eggs and vanilla. Overlap in the chocolate chips last. (On the off chance that you'd like, you can save 1/4 cup of the chocolate chips to add on top.)

4. Scoop the player equally into the biscuit cups, filling practically full. On the off chance that you held some chocolate contributes the past advance, sprinkle them on top and press delicately into the player.

5. Bake it for 25 min., until the tops are brilliant and an embedded toothpick tells the truth.

NUTRITION INFORMATION
Calories233 | Fat20g | Protein10g | Total Carbs10g | Net Carbs5g | Fiber5g | Sugar0g

CHIP CHOCOLATE LOW-CARB PALEO ZUCCHINI MUFFINS RECIPE

For the most delightful low carb zucchini biscuits or paleo zucchini biscuits, attempt this chocolate chip zucchini biscuits formula with coconut flour! It's sans sugar, keto, sans nut, and without dairy.

Course: Breakfast, Dessert

Cooking: American

Prep Time: 10 minutes

Cook Time: 35 minutes

Total Time: 45 minutes

Serving size: 1 biscuit

INGREDIENTS
3/4 cup Coconut flour
1/2 cup Erythritol
2 tsp without gluten Preparing powder
1/4 tsp Sea salt
8 oz Zucchini (destroyed/ground, around 2 cups)

6 huge Egg

1/2 tsp Vanilla concentrate

2/3 cup Ghee (estimated strong, at that point liquefied; can likewise utilize without dairy spread enhanced coconut oil)

1/2 cup sans sugar dim chocolate chips

DIRECTIONS

1. Preheat the broiler to 350 degrees F (177 degrees C). Line a biscuit skillet with 12 material paper liners.

2. In an enormous bowl, mix together the coconut flour, sugar, heating powder, and ocean salt.

3. Add the destroyed zucchini, eggs, and vanilla. Mix together until joined. Include the softened coconut oil and mix again until smooth.

4. Fold in the chocolate chips. Let the player sit for 5 minutes to thicken.

5. Divide the hitter among the material liners, filling them right to the top. Whenever wanted, you can spot the tops with more chocolate chips.

6. Bake for around 35 minutes, until brilliant and firm on top. Cool to room temperature in the dish, at that point on a wire rack. You can eat them warm, yet the surface is better in the event that you let them cool first.

NUTRITION INFORMATION
Calories181 | Fat15g | Protein5g | Total Carbs8g | Net Carbs4g | Fiber4g | Sugar1g

LOW CARB-CHOCOLATE CHIP PEANUT BUTTER PROTEIN COOKIES RECIPE

This easy chocolate chip nutty spread protein Cookies formula is so chewy. Only the 6 ingredients, 1 bowl, and 10 minutes Prep for delectable, flourless low carb-protein Cookies. They're normally without gluten.

Course: Breakfast, Dessert

Cooking: American

Calories: 118 kcal

Prep Time: 10 minutes

Cook Time: 20 minutes

Total Time: 30 minutes

Serving size: 1 treat

INGREDIENTS
1/3 cup Vital Proteins Collagen Peptides
1/2 cup Erythritol (or any granulated sugar)
1/4 tsp Sea salt
1 cup Peanut margarine (no sugar included)
2 enormous Eggs
1 tsp Vanilla concentrate
1/3 cup sans sugar dim chocolate chips

DIRECTIONS
1. Preheat the broiler to 350 degrees F (177 degrees C). Line a heating sheet with material paper.

2. In a huge bowl, mix together the collagen, sugar, and ocean salt.

3. Add the egg and rush at the edge of the bowl to blend the yolk and white, before blending in with the dry ingredients. Include the nutty spread and vanilla, and mix until smooth.

4. Fold in the chocolate chips.

5. Scoop the treat batter utilizing a medium treat scoop, and press the mixture into it before discharging onto the lined Preparing sheet. Squash the treat mixture balls with the

palm of your hand or the base of a wet glass, to around 1/4 in (~1/2 cm) thickness.

6. Bake this recipes for 16-20 min., until the Cookies are semi-firm and not clingy on top. Cool Totally to solidify more.

NUTRITION INFORMATION
Calories118 | Fat8g | Protein7g | Total Carbs4g| Net Carbs2g | Fiber2g | Sugar0g

CHOCOLATE PEANUT AND BUTTER LOW CARB SMOOTHIE RECIPE

This keto chocolate nutty spread smoothie formula will be one of your fave healthy low carb smoothies. So rich, and Prepared in a short time with 5 ingredients!

Course: Breakfast, Drinks

Cooking: American

Calories: 435 kcal

Prep Time: 5 minutes

Total Time: 5 minutes

Servings: 1 cup each

INGREDIENTS
1/4 cup Peanut spread (rich)
3 tbsp Cocoa powder
1 cup of heavy cream (or coconut cream for without dairy or veggie lover)
1 1/2 cup unsweetened almond milk (ordinary or vanilla)
6 tbsp Powdered erythritol (to taste)

1/8 tsp Sea salt (discretionary)

DIRECTIONS
1. Combine all ingredients in a blender.

2. Puree until smooth. Modify sugar to taste whenever wanted.

NUTRITION INFORMATION
Calories435 | Fat41g | Protein9g | Total Carbs10g | Net Carbs6g | Fiber4g | Sugar3g

FATHEAD KETO CINNAMON ROLLS RECIPE - QUICK and EASY

Everybody cherishes these keto cinnamon rolls! Just 40 minutes to make, with basic ingredients (no exceptional flour!), and they're totally tasty. For a stunning low carb dessert or keto breakfast, attempt this fathead cinnamon moves formula.

Course: Breakfast, Dessert

Food: American

Calories: 321 kcal

Prep Time: 20 minutes

Cook Time: 20 minutes

Total Time: 40 minutes

Serving size: 1 cinnamon roll

INGREDIENTS
2 cup Macadamia nuts (10 oz)
1/4 cup Erythritol
1 tbsp sans gluten heating powder

2 enormous Egg
1 tsp Vanilla concentrate (discretionary)
4 cup Mozzarella cheddar (destroyed)
4 oz Cream cheddar

Filling
1/4 cup Butter (softened)
1/2 cup Erythritol
2 tbsp Cinnamon

Icing
1/3 cup sans sugar cream cheddar icing
1 tbsp of almond milk (or any milk of decision)

DIRECTIONS
1. Put the macadamia nuts into a food processor fitted with a S blade sharp edge. Heartbeat just until the nuts arrive at a fine, brittle consistency, without huge pieces. Make a point to beat, don't leave the food processor running, to attempt to make flour and not nut margarine. Scratch the sides varying. The nuts may, in any case, start to shape nut margarine a bit, however, attempt to stay away from however much as could be expected.

2. Add the erythritol and heating powder. Heartbeat a few times, just until blended.

3. Add the eggs and vanilla. Heartbeat several times once more, just until blended.

4. Heat the mozzarella and cream cheddar in the microwave for around 2 minutes, blending part of the way through and toward the end, or on the stove in a twofold evaporator, until easy to mix. Mix until smooth.

5. Add the cheddar blend to the food processor. Push the cheddar blend down into the nut/egg blend. Heartbeat/puree until uniform mixture structures, scratching down the sides vary. If you experience difficulty getting it to blend, you can massage a little with a spatula and afterwards beat some more.

6. Refrigerate the batter directly in the food processor for around 30-an hour, until the top is firm and not clingy.

7. Meanwhile, preheat the stove to 375 degrees F (191 degrees C). Line a 9x13 in

(23x33 cm) heating container with material paper.

8. Take the batter out onto an enormous bit of material paper (not the one on the heating sheet). It will, in any case, be genuinely clingy. Utilize a tad of the softened margarine on your hands to forestall staying as you spread it into a square shape.

9. Brush the mixture square shape with the majority of the staying softened margarine, leaving aside around 1-2 tablespoons. Mix together the erythritol and cinnamon for the filling. Sprinkle the blend uniformly over the square shape.

10. Oil your hands again with the softened spread. Beginning from a long side of the square shape, fold up the mixture into a log. As you come, oil the underside of the log as you strip it away from the material underneath during rolling. (This is to forestall breaking and staying.)

11. Slice the sign into 1 in (2.5 cm) thick cuts, which will look like pinwheels. Spot the pinwheels level onto the lined Preparing

dish, practically contacting however not exactly.

12. Bake for around 25 minutes, until the keto cinnamon rolls are brilliant on top. Cool for in any event 20 minutes, until firm.

13. Meanwhile, making the icing. Beat almond milk into the icing a tablespoon at once, until the icing is sufficiently slender to shower. When the keto cinnamon rolls are sufficiently firm, sprinkle the icing over them.

NUTRITION INFORMATION
Calories321 | Fat29.5g | Protein11g | Total Carbs5g | Net Carbs3g | Fiber2g | Sugar1g

EASY KETO ALMOND FLOUR PANCAKES RECIPE

These soft almond flour hotcakes are so easy to make! Only a couple of basic ingredients required. You're going to cherish this easy keto almond flour hotcake formula. They're paleo, as well!

Course: Breakfast, Main Course

Cooking: American

Calories: 261 kcal

Prep Time: 5 minutes

Cook Time: 15 minutes

Total Time: 20 minutes

Serving size: 3-inch flapjacks

INGREDIENTS
1 cup Blanched almond flour
2 tbsp Erythritol (or any sugar; use coconut sugar for paleo)
1 tsp sans gluten heating powder

1/8 tsp Sea salt

2 eggs

1/3 cup of unsweetened almond milk (or any milk of decision)

2 tbsp Avocado oil (or any nonpartisan oil of decision; in addition to additional for singing)

1 tsp Vanilla concentrate (discretionary)

DIRECTIONS

1. Mix the ingredients together in a can until smooth.

2. Preheat an oiled dish on the stove at medium-low warmth. Pour circles of player onto the dish, 1/8 cup (30 mL) at once for 3 in (8 cm) flapjacks. Spread and Cook around 1/2 to 2 minutes, until bubbles begin to frame on the edges. Flip and Cook one more moment or two, until seared on the opposite side.

3. Repeat with the rest of the hitter.

NUTRITION INFORMATION

Calories261 | Fat23g | Protein9g | Total Carbs6g | Net Carbs4g | Fiber2g | Sugar1g

RECIPES FOR LUNCH AND DINNER

LOW CARB KETO CABBAGE ROLLS RECIPE WITHOUT RICE

Perceive how to make cabbage moves without rice that are similarly as delightful! This easy low carb keto cabbage moves formula is comfort food reconsidered.

Course: Main Course

Food: Polish

Calories: 321 kcal

Prep Time: 25 minutes

Cook Time: 60 minutes

Total Time: 1 hour 25 minutes

Serving size: 2 cabbage rolls

INGREDIENTS

1 head Cabbage
1 lb ground hamburger
1 14.5-oz can Diced tomatoes (depleted)
1 enormous Egg
4 cloves Garlic (minced)
2 tsp Italian flavouring
1 tsp Sea salt
1/4 tsp Black pepper
1 cup Cauliflower rice
1 15-oz would tomato be able to sauce

DIRECTIONS

1. Preheat the broiler to 350 degrees F (177 degrees C).

2. Bring an enormous pot of water to a bubble. Include the head of cabbage into the bubbling water, drenching completely. Bubble for 5-8 minutes, just until the leaves are sufficiently delicate to twist. They will turn brilliant green, and the external leaves may fall off, which is alright and you can angle them out.

3. Remove the cabbage from the bubbling water. Put aside to cool. Leave the boiling

water in the pot until further notice, and you may require it again later when stripping the cabbage leaves.

4. Meanwhile, pan sears the cauliflower rice for a couple of moments as per the guidelines here.

5. In an enormous bowl, join the ground hamburger, diced tomatoes, egg, minced garlic, Italian flavouring, ocean salt, and dark pepper. Blend until simply consolidated, yet don't over-blend—overlap in the cooked cauliflower rice. Put in a safe spot.

6. Spread the large part of the tomato sauce in an enormous rectangular or oval clay heating dish. Put in a safe spot.

7. Carefully strip the leaves from the cabbage. To do this, flip cabbage over such a centre side is up, and cut the leaves individually from the centre, at that point cautiously strip (they are delicate). Rather than stripping leaves back, slide your fingers between the layers of cabbage to discharge them. The leaves outwardly will be delicate and simpler to strip, yet inside they might be

firmer. In the event that they are excessively firm and fresh to twist, you can restore the incompletely stripped cabbage to bubbling water for a couple more minutes to mollify more.

8. Cut the thick rib from the focal point of each cabbage leaf, cutting in a "V" shape. Spot 1/3 cup (67 grams) hamburger blend into a log shape toward one side of a cabbage leaf. Overlay in the sides, at that point, move up, similar to a burrito. Spot the cabbage move, crease side down, into the heating dish over the sauce. Rehash to make 12 cabbage rolls. (In the event that the inward leaves are excessively little, you may need to utilize two to cover them to fit the filling.)

9. Spread the preparing dish firmly with foil. Bake for 60 minutes, or until the meat is Cooked through.

NUTRITION INFORMATION

Calories321 | Fat18g | Protein25g | Total Carbs15g | Net Carbs10g | Fiber5g | Sugar7g

KETO BUFFALO CHICKEN SPAGHETTI SQUASH CASSEROLE RECIPE

You need only 6 straightforward ingredients for keto bison chicken spaghetti squash goulash. Make this gooey spaghetti squash meal formula for a healthy, encouraging meal today around evening time!

Course: Main Course

Food: Dinner

Calories: 301 kcal

Prep Time: 15 minutes

Cook Time: 40 minutes

Total Time: 55 minutes

Serving size: 1/3 cup or 1/6 of formula

INGREDIENTS

1 medium Spaghetti squash

1 cup Blue cheddar dressing (in addition to additional for garnish)

1/4 cup Buffalo sauce (will be mellow; can add more to taste)

4 oz Cream cheddar (mellowed)

2 cups Shredded chicken (Cooked)

1 cup cheddar (destroyed)

Green onions (discretionary, for garnish)

DIRECTIONS

1. Preheat the broiler to 400 degrees F (204 degrees C).

2. Use a blade to jab a couple of openings everywhere throughout the spaghetti squash. Spot onto a heating sheet and prepare for 30-40 minutes, until a blade goes in with almost no opposition. Expel from the stove (leave it on) and put in a safe spot.

3. Meanwhile, in an enormous bowl, mix together the blue cheddar dressing, wild ox sauce, and cream cheddar. Mix in the destroyed chicken.

4. Cut the spaghetti squash into equal parts and utilize a spoon to scoop out the seeds. Utilize a fork to discharge the strands into the bowl with the chicken blend. Mix together.

5. Transfer the goulash blend to an enormous meal dish (12x8" oval dish, 2.4 qt.). Top with destroyed cheddar. Spot in the broiler for 10 minutes, until the cheddar dissolves.

6. If wanted, shower the top with extra blue cheddar dressing and sprinkle with green onions.

NUTRITION INFORMATION
Calories301 | Fat20g | Protein19g | Total Carbs14g | Net Carbs12g | Fiber2g | Sugar6g

CHIPOTLE BEEF BARBACOA RECIPE (SLOW COOKER/CROCKPOT)

The best Crock Pot barbacoa ever! On the off chance that you love barbacoa meat, you need to attempt this copycat Chipotle barbacoa formula in a slow Cooker. It's healthy, easy, low carb, and self-destruct tastily.

Course: Main Course

Food: American

Calories: 242 kcal

Prep Time: 10 minutes

Cook Time: 4 hours

Total Time: 4 hours 10 minutes

Serving size: 1/3 lb, or 1/9 whole formula

INGREDIENTS

3 lb Beef brisket or throw broil (cut and cut into 2-inch lumps)

1/2 cup Beef soup (or chicken stock)

2 medium Chipotle chiles in adobo (counting the sauce, around 4 tsp)

5 cloves Garlic (minced)

2 tbsp Apple juice vinegar

2 tbsp Lime juice

1 tbsp dried oregano

2 tsp Cumin

2 tsp Sea salt

1 tsp Black pepper

1/2 tsp Ground cloves (discretionary)

2 entire Bay leaf

DIRECTIONS

1. Combine the soup, chipotle chiles in adobo sauce, garlic, apple juice vinegar, lime juice, dried oregano, cumin, ocean salt, dark pepper, and ground cloves in a blender (everything with the exception of the hamburger and cove leaves). Puree until smooth.

2. Place the hamburger lumps in the slow Cooker. Pour the pureed blend from the

blender on top. Include the (entire) cove leaves.

3. Cook for 4-6 hrs. on high temp. or 8-10 hrs. on low, until the meat is self-destructed delicate.

4. Remove the straight leaves. Shred the meat utilizing two forks and mix into the juices. Spread and rest for 5-10 minutes to allow the meat to ingest much more flavour. Utilize an opened spoon to serve.

NUTRITION INFORMATION
Calories242 | Fat11g | Protein32g | Total Carbs2g | Net Carbs1g | Fiber1g | Sugar0.3g

FIRM BAKED CHICKEN LEGS DRUMSTICKS RECIPE

This 10-minute-Prep easy stove broiled chicken drumsticks formula will make super firm prepared chicken legs that turn out splendidly inevitably! It's the main guide for how to prepare chicken legs you'll ever require.

Course: Main Course

Food: American

Calories: 236 kcal

Prep Time: 10 minutes

Cook Time: 40 minutes

Total Time: 50 minutes

Serving size: 1 drumstick

INGREDIENTS
6 medium chicken drumsticks (~1 1/2 lb)
1/4 cup butter (softened)
1/2 tsp smoked paprika

1/2 tsp Garlic powde
1/2 tsp Sea salt
1/4 tsp Black pepper

DIRECTIONS

1. Preheat the broiler to 425 degrees F (218 degrees C). Line a heating sheet with foil and spot a broiler-safe rack on top.

2. Organize the chicken legs on the rack.

3. Brush the chicken drumsticks with dissolved margarine—season with smoked paprika, garlic powder, salt and pepper.

4. Bake the chicken legs in the stove for 25 minutes. Flip and heat for another 10-20 minutes, until the inner temperature comes to in any event 165 degrees F (74 degrees C).

NUTRITION INFORMATION
Calories236 | Fat16g | Protein22g | Total Carbs0g | Net Carbs0g | Fiber0g | Sugar0g

ITALIAN STUFFED ARTICHOKES RECIPE WITH SAUSAGE

Figure out how to make stuffed artichokes in the broiler with bit by bit pictures! This prepared Italian stuffed artichokes formula makes a tasty low carb meal or hors d'oeuvre.

Course: Main Course

Cooking: Italian

Calories: 604 kcal

Prep Time: 20 minutes

Cook Time: 55 minutes

Total Time: 1 hour 15 minutes

Serving size: 1 stuffed artichoke*

INGREDIENTS

Artichokes:

4 huge Ocean Mist Farms Artichokes

2 tbsp Lemon juice

2 tbsp Olive oil

2 tbsp Grated Parmesan cheddar (separated)

Filling:

1 lb Ground Italian Sausage

4 cloves Garlic (minced)

2 tsp Italian flavouring

1/2 cup Grated Parmesan cheddar (separated)

DIRECTIONS

1. Cut about an inch off the highest points of the artichokes and remove the stems to make a level base. Use kitchen shears to trim the sharp warns the leaves.

2. Bring a huge pot of saltwater to a bubble. Include the artichokes and spot a warmth safe dish on them to keep them submerged in the water—bubble for 15 minutes. Evacuate and put aside topsy turvy to deplete and cool.

3. Meanwhile, preheat the broiler to 375 degrees F (190 degrees C).

4. In an enormous bowl, combine the Italian hotdog, minced garlic, Italian flavouring and 1/2 cup (50 grams) ground parmesan, until simply joined. Don't over-blend.

5. Once the artichokes are sufficiently cool to deal with, dry them with paper towels, tenderly pry open the middle leaves, and utilize a spoon with a curving movement to scoop out the fluffy gag inside. Spot the artichokes into a stoneware heating dish, looking up.

6. Drizzle the artichokes done with lemon juice and olive oil, including the tops and sides.

7. Stuff every artichoke with the frankfurter blend, ensuring you get some between all the leaves and in the middle. Sprinkle the artichokes with the staying 2 tablespoons (30 grams) ground parmesan.

8. Cover the heating dish with foil. Prepare for 40-50 minutes, until the hotdog is Cooked through (to an interior temperature of 165 degrees F (74 degrees C)) and the external leaves are easy to expel.

9. Remove the foil. Set the stove to sear and put the stuffed artichokes under the oven for two or three minutes to dark-coloured the cheddar.

*Nutrition data is expected for a full, filling meal. On the off chance that you are viewing carbs or calories, a large portion of a stuffed artichoke would, in any case, be a bounty for a serving. Serving size could be 1/8 or 1/4 of the stuffed artichoke as an hors d'oeuvre.

NUTRITION INFORMATION
Calories604 | Fat47g | Protein28g | Total Carbs21g | Net Carbs12g | Fiber9g | Sugar2g

LOW CARB KETO CHEESY TACO SKILLET RECIPE

A keto mushy taco skillet formula in only 25 minutes, with 7 basic ingredients! This easy hamburger taco skillet dinner is ideal for occupied weeknights.

Course: Main Course

Food: Mexican

Calories: 547 kcal

Cook Time: 25 minutes

Total Time: 25 minutes

Serving size: 1/2 cups, or 1/4 whole skillet*

*This is a liberal serving size. Contingent upon your requirements, you could separate the skillet into 6 servings rather than 4 for littler segments and 9g net carbs per serving.

INGREDIENTS

1 lb ground hamburger
2 tbsp Taco flavouring
1/2 cup Water
1/2 enormous Onion (diced)
3 enormous Bell peppers (cut into 1-inch strips)
1 14.5-oz can Dice tomatoes (depleted well)
1 cup Mexican cheddar mix (destroyed)
1/4 cup Green onions (cut)

DIRECTIONS

1. Heat a skillet over medium-high warmth. Include ground hamburger and cook around 10 minutes, breaking separated the meat with a spatula or spoon, until seared.

2. Add the taco flavouring and water. Cook for 2-3 minutes, until the additional water, is ingested or vanishes.

3. Reduce warmth to medium. Include the onions and ringer peppers. Cook for 5-10 minutes, until onions are delicate and translucent.

4. Add the diced tomatoes. Stew for a couple of moments, until hot and any additional dampness vanishes.

5. Reduce warmth to low. Sprinkle destroyed cheddar on top. Spread with a cover and warmth just until the cheddar dissolves. Expel from warmth and top with green onions.

NUTRITION INFORMATION
Calories547 | Fat35g | Protein41g | Total Carbs17g | Net Carbs12g | Fiber5g | Sugar9g

SMOTHERED PORK CHOPS RECIPE WITH ONION GRAVY

A tasty, easy heated covered pork cleaves formula with onion sauce! Perceive how to make the juiciest covered pork slashes in the broiler, with only 7 ingredients.

Course: Main Course

Food: American

Calories: 541 kcal

Prep Time: 10 minutes

Cook Time: 50 minutes

Total Time: 60 minutes

Serving size: 1 pork slash with gravy*

*Nutrition data is for huge, 8-ounce pork slashes. Contingent upon what you're serving them with, it might bode well to slice the serving size down the middle to 4 ounces.

INGREDIENTS
4 8-oz Boneless pork cleaves
1 tsp Sea salt
1/4 tsp Black pepper
2 tbsp Olive oil
1 enormous Onion (cut into slender half moons)
2 cloves of Garlic (minced)
1 cup of Chicken juices
1.5 oz of Cream cheddar (cut into little lumps)

DIRECTIONS
1. Season the pork slashes on the two sides with ocean salt, garlic powder, onion powder, and pepper.

2. Heat the olive oil in a dutch broiler over medium-high warmth. Include the pork hacks and burn on the two sides, around 3 minutes for each side without moving, until seared. Move the pork slashes to a plate and put in a safe spot.

3. Reduce warmth to medium-low or medium. Utilizing a similar dutch broiler, saute the cut onions for 15-20 minutes, until caramelized.

4. Once the onions are caramelized, preheat the stove to 375 degrees F (190 degrees C).

5. Saute for about a moment, until fragrant.

6. Add the chicken soup to the dutch broiler—Scratch any caramelized bits from the base of the skillet. Bring to a delicate bubble, at that point stew for around 2-3 minutes, until it gets thicker and the volume is decreased by at any rate 1/4.

7. Remove from heat. Include the cream cheddar. Mix in the cream cheddar until it dissolves into the sauce.

8. Return the pork hacks to the dutch broiler and spoon the sauce and onions over them. Spread with the cover and prepare for 20-25 minutes, until cooked through.

NUTRITION INFORMATION
Calories541 | Fat35g | Protein48g | Total Carbs5g | Net Carbs4g | Fiber1g | Sugar2g

LOW CARB KETO TURKEY MEATLOAF RECIPE

The entire family will adore this keto turkey meatloaf formula! Low carb bacon-wrapped turkey meatloaf is delightful, delicious, and takes only 10 minutes to Prep.

Course Main: Course

Food: American

Calories: 241 kcal

Prep Time: 10 minutes

Cook Time: 50 minutes

Total Time: 60 minutes

Serving size: 1 3/4-inch cut, or 1/12 whole meatloaf

INGREDIENTS
Turkey Meatloaf:
2 lb ground turkey
1/2 enormous Onion (cleaved finely)
6 cloves Garlic (minced)

1/3 cup Tomato sauce
2 tsp Italian flavouring
1 1/2 tsp Sea salt
 1/4 tsp Black pepper
1/2 cup Blanched almond flour
2 enormous Eggs

Beating:
10 cuts Bacon
1/4 cup sans sugar BBQ sauce

DIRECTIONS
1. Preheat the broiler to 350 degrees F (177 degrees C). Line a Preparing sheet with foil or material paper.

2. In an enormous bowl, consolidate all turkey meatloaf ingredients. Blend until simply consolidated - don't over blend.

3. Form the ground turkey blend into a 10x6 inch portion on the lined heating sheet.

4. Arrange the bacon cuts in a solitary layer on the meatloaf, going over the short way, and fold the closures underneath the sides of the meatloaf.

5. Bake for 30 minutes.

6. Spread the BBQ sauce and sides of the turkey meatloaf. Come back to the broiler and heat for 20-35 additional minutes, until cooked through and inner temperature arrives at 160 degrees F (71 degrees C). (Time will shift contingent upon the thickness of the portion.) If wanted, place under the grill for a couple of moments to fresh up the bacon.

7. Rest for 10 minutes before cutting utilizing a serrated blade.

NUTRITION INFORMATION
Calories241 | Fat17g | Protein19g | Total Carbs4g | Net Carbs3g | Fiber1g | Sugar 1g

LOW CARB KETO CABBAGE ROLLS RECIPE WITHOUT RICE

Perceive how to make cabbage moves without rice that are similarly as flavorful! This easy, whole30, low carb keto cabbage moves formula is comfort food reconsidered.

Course: Main Course

Cooking: Polish

Calories: 321 kcal

Prep Time: 25 minutes

Cook Time: 60 minutes

Total Time: 1 hour 25 minutes

Servings

INGREDIENTS

1 head Cabbage

1 lb ground hamburger

1 14.5-oz can Diced tomatoes (depleted)

1 enormous Egg

4 cloves Garlic (minced)

2 tsp Italian flavouring

1 tsp Sea salt

1/4 tsp Black pepper

1 cup Cauliflower rice

1 15-oz would tomato be able to sauce

DIRECTIONS

1. Preheat the broiler to 350 degrees F (177 degrees C).

2. Bring an enormous pot of water to a bubble. Include the head of cabbage into the bubbling water, inundating completely. Bubble for 5-8 minutes, just until the leaves are sufficiently delicate to twist. They will turn brilliant green, and the external leaves may fall off, which is alright and you can angle them out.

3. Remove the cabbage from the bubbling water. Put aside to cool. Leave the heated water in the pot until further notice, and you

may require it again later when stripping the cabbage leaves.

4. Meanwhile, pan sears the cauliflower rice for a couple of moments as per the guidelines here.

5. In an enormous bowl, join the ground hamburger, diced tomatoes, egg, minced garlic, Italian flavouring, ocean salt, and dark pepper. Blend until simply joined, yet don't over-blend—crease in the Cooked cauliflower rice. Put in a safe spot.

6. Spread part of the tomato sauce in an enormous rectangular or oval artistic heating dish. Put in a safe spot.

7. Carefully strip the leaves from the cabbage. To do this, flip cabbage over such a centre side is up, and cut the leaves individually from the centre, at that point cautiously strip (they are delicate). Rather than stripping leaves back, slide your fingers between the layers of cabbage to discharge them. The leaves outwardly will be delicate and simpler to strip, however inside they might be firmer. In the event that they are excessively firm and fresh to twist, you can

restore the somewhat stripped cabbage to bubbling water for a couple more minutes to mollify more.

8. Cut the thick rib from the focal point of each cabbage leaf, cutting in a "V" shape. Spot 1/3 cup (67 grams) meat blend into a log shape toward one side of a cabbage leaf. Overlay in the sides, at that point, move up, similar to a burrito. Spot the cabbage move, crease side down, into the preparing dish over the sauce. Rehash to make 12 cabbage rolls. (In the event that the inward leaves are excessively little, you may need to utilize two to cover them to fit the filling.)

9. Spread the preparing dish firmly with foil—Bake for 60 minutes, or until the hamburger is cooked through.

NUTRITION INFORMATION
 Calories321 | Fat18g | Protein25g | Total Carbs15g | Net Carbs10g | Fiber5g | Sugar7g

KETO MEXICAN CHEESE AND CHICKEN STUFFED POBLANO PEPPERS RECIPE

Perceive how to make Mexican keto stuffed poblano peppers with basic ingredients, in only 30 minutes! This mushy chicken stuffed poblano peppers formula is loaded with taco flavours.

Course: dinner

Cooking: Mexican

Calories: 216 kcal

Prep Time: 5 minutes

Cook Time: 20 minutes

Total Time: 25 minutes

Serving size: 1 stuffed pepper

INGREDIENTS
3 huge Poblano peppers
1 tbsp Butter
2 cloves Garlic (minced)

2 cups shredded chicken

1 14.5-oz can Diced tomatoes (NOT depleted)

2 tbsp Taco flavouring

3 oz Cream cheddar (cubed)

3/4 cup cheddar (destroyed)

Cilantro (discretionary, for fixing)

DIRECTIONS

1. Pre-heat the stove to 350 degrees F (177 degrees C).

2. Cut the peppers down the middle and evacuate the seeds. Spot them onto a lined Preparing sheet. Put in a safe spot.

3. In a skillet over medium warmth, liquefy the margarine. Include the garlic and saute for around 30 seconds, until fragrant.

4. Add the destroyed chicken, diced tomatoes (with fluid), and taco flavouring. Heat the stew for 3-5 minutes, until the additional fluid is ingested into the chicken.

5. Reduce warmth to low. Mix in the cream cheddar, squeezing with the rear of a spoon or spatula to assist it with blending in, until softened and smooth.

6. Stuff it into the poblano peppers and spot, open side up, back onto the heating sheet. Sprinkle destroyed cheddar on each pepper half, around 2 tablespoons (28 grams) each.

7. Bake for 15-20 minutes, until peppers are delicate and cheddar is softened. Embellishment with crisp cilantro whenever wanted.

NUTRITION INFORMATION
Calories216 | Fat15g | Protein16g | Total Carbs6g | Net Carbs4g | Fiber2g | Sugar3g

HALIBUT RECIPE WITH LEMON BUTTER SAUCE

This dish singed halibut formula with lemon margarine sauce takes only 20 minutes... which you'd never surmise with how extravagant seared halibut looks. I'll tell you the best way to container burn halibut, in addition to how to make the ideal sauce for halibut.

Course: dinner, Main Course

Cooking: American

Calories: 513 kcal

Prep Time: 5 minutes

Cook Time: 10 minutes

Total Time: 15 minutes

Serving size: 1 halibut filet + 2 tbsp lemon margarine sauce

INGREDIENTS

4 6-oz of Halibut fillets (1.5 lb Total)
1/2 tsp of Garlic powder
1/2 tsp of Paprika
1 tsp of Sea salt
1/4 tsp of Black pepper
2 tbsp of Olive oil

Lemon spread sauce:
1/2 cup Salted spread
1 medium Lemon (cut down the middle)

DIRECTIONS

1. Use paper towels to pat the halibut filets totally dry - this will guarantee in any event, sautéing. Season the fish on the two sides with garlic powder, paprika, ocean salt, and dark pepper. Put in a safe spot.

2. Heat the olive oil in an enormous skillet over medium-high warmth for 2 minutes.

3. Add the fish filets in a solitary layer (you can do it in clumps if all the fish won't fit in a solitary layer). Burn, without moving, for 3-4 minutes, until the edges of the fish are misty.

4. Remove the fish from the container and spread firmly with foil to keep warm.

5. Reduce warmth to medium-low. Add the spread to a similar dish. Hang tight for it to dissolve, at that point heat for 2-3 minutes, mixing every so often, until the margarine is cooked and smells nutty.

6. Use the Zulay Kitchen Lemon Squeezer to crush all the juice from the two parts of the lemon into the container. Bring to a stew, at that point diminish warmth and stew for around 3-4 minutes, frequently mixing, until the volume is decreased considerably. The lemon margarine sauce will, in any case, be slender.

7. Drizzle a little lemon margarine sauce over each serving plate. Spot the skillet burned halibut filets over the sauce, at that point shower more sauce on top.

NUTRITION INFORMATION
Calories513 | Fat35g | Protein47g | Total Carbs3g | Net Carbs2g | Fiber1g | Sugar1g

LOW CARB KETO BUFFALO CHICKEN MEATBALLS RECIPE

Perceive how to make wild ox chicken meatballs with only 6 ingredients! This easy low carb keto bison chicken meatballs formula is a mashup of wings + meatballs, with just 10 minutes Prep.

Course: Appetizer, Main Course

Cooking: American

Calories: 230 kcal

Prep Time: 10 minutes

Cook Time: 15 minutes

Total Time: 25 minutes

Serving size: 4 meatballs

INGREDIENTS

1 1/2 lb of ground chicken

1/4 cup of egg whites (2 medium egg whites)

1/2 cup of Blue cheddar (disintegrated)

1/2 cup of green onions (hacked)

1/2 cup of buffalo sauce

1 tbsp of olive oil

DIRECTIONS

1. Preheat the stove to 400 degrees F (204 degrees C). Line a heating sheet with material paper or a silicone tangle.

2. Combine the ground chicken, egg whites, blue cheddar, scallions, and 3/4 of the cayenne pepper sauce in a bowl. Structure into 1 in (2.5 cm) balls and spot on the lined Preparing sheet. Prepare for 12-15 minutes, until scarcely done.

3. Meanwhile, whisk together the rest of the cayenne pepper sauce with the olive oil.

4. Drain the liquid discharged by the meatballs and move them to a spotless sheet of material paper (still on the heating sheet). Sprinkle a limited quantity of the cayenne,

olive oil blend over every meatball—heat for 2-3 minutes.

NUTRITION INFORMATION
Calories230 | Fat15g | Protein23g | Total Carbs1g | Net Carbs0g | Fiber1g | Sugar1g

THE CROCKPOT WHOLE CHICKEN WITH GARLIC HERB & BUTTER

this crock-pot entire chicken formula is easy, and slow cooker entire chicken turns out juicy without fail! only 15 minutes to prep.

Course: dinner

Food: American

Calories: 394 kcal

Prep Time: 15 minutes

Cook Time: 3 hours

Resting Time: 10 minutes

Total Time: 3 hours 15 minutes

INGREDIENTS
4 sprigs Fresh rosemary (isolated)
12 sprigs Fresh thyme (isolated)
6 tbsp Butter (relaxed)
1 head Garlic (4 cloves minced, staying ones
stripped and entirety)
2 tsp Fresh parsley (slashed)
2 tsp Sea salt
1/2 tsp Paprika
1/2 tsp Black pepper
1 5-lb Whole chicken
1 enormous Yellow onion (cut into huge,
thick cuts)

DIRECTIONS
1. Remove the leaves from a large portion of
the rosemary (2 sprigs) and a large portion
of the thyme (6 sprigs). (Put the staying
entire sprigs in a safe spot.) Chop the
rosemary finely.

2. In a little bowl, pound together the
margarine, 4 cloves minced garlic, hacked

rosemary, cleaved thyme, slashed parsley, salt, paprika, and pepper. Put in a safe spot.

3. Use the paper-towels to pat the chicken , with the goal that the herb spread sticks better. (For food wellbeing reasons, it's better NOT to flush it.)

4. Grease the base of the Crock-Pot Cook and carry slow cooker with more margarine. Spot the onion pieces inside. Put the entire chicken, bosom side up, on the onions.

5. Starting from the hole side of the chicken, delicately embed your hands underneath the skin to isolate the skin from the meat, including the bosom, thighs and legs. Be mindful so as not to tear the skin it.

6. Use your hands to rub a large portion of the garlic herb spread all over underneath the skin. Rub the rest of the margarine everywhere throughout the top and sides of the chicken. (On the off chance that your margarine isn't too delicate, first mellow it by setting it into a little bowl longer than the second bowl of warm water. Soft margarine will be simpler to spread!)

7. Stuff the staying entire garlic cloves (6-10 cloves), staying 2 entire rosemary sprigs, and staying 6 entire thyme sprigs inside the chicken pit. Tie the legs together with kitchen twine. In the event that essential, reposition the chicken and onions so the chicken is perched on top and the onions are raising the chicken.

8. Cover the Crock-Pot Cooker and Cook for 5-8 hrs on Low or 3-5 hours on High, until the inward temperature comes to at any rate 160 degrees (72 degrees C) inside (it will rise another 5 degrees during searing and resting). On the off chance that your garlic margarine didn't spread well in the first place, you can lift the top about an hour into Cooking and utilize a cake brush to spread the herb margarine all the more equitably ridiculous and sides of the chicken. (Try not to utilize dissolved margarine from the earliest starting point since it will all dribble off the cool chicken.)

9. When the chicken is done, dispose of the onions however spare the fluid below, which you can use as chicken soup in recipes!

10. Optional advance for fresh skin: toward the end, preheat the oven and spot the rack close to it, with simply enough space for the chicken to fit underneath. Move the chicken to a preparing dish or cooking container and sear for 4-6 minutes, until caramelized.

NUTRITION INFORMATION
Calories394 | Fat30g | Protein24g | Total Carbs4g | Net Carbs4g | Fiber0g | Sugar1g

CROCKPOT SLOW COOKER TURKEY BREAST RECIPE

Figure out how to cook a turkey bosom to be superbly juicy with this easy Crock-Pot slow Cooker turkey bosom formula! Only 10 minutes to prep, at that point the bone-in turkey bosom cooks itself.

Course: Main Course

Cooking: American

Calories: 317 kcal

Prep Time: 10 minutes

Cook Time: 4 hours

Total Time: 4 hours 10 minutes

Serving size: ~6-8 oz Cooked turkey, or 1/6 of the whole formula

* Onion is excluded from nutrition data since it's there for seasoning and lifting the turkey meat and is ordinarily disposed of. Serving size weight is a consumable bit, excluding bones.

INGREDIENTS

7-lb Bone-in turkey bosom (2 parts joined at the bosom bone)

1/4 cup Butter (mellowed; in addition to additional for lubing the slow cooker)

2 tsp Sea salt

1/2 tsp Black pepper

4 cloves garlic (minced)

2 tsp fresh rosemary

2 tsp fresh thyme

2 tsp fresh parsley

1/2 tsp Paprika

1 huge Yellow onion (cut into enormous, thick cuts)

1/2 cup Chicken juices

DIRECTIONS

1. In a little bowl, pound together the spread, salt, pepper, garlic, rosemary, thyme, parsley, and paprika.

2. Use the paper-towels to pat the turkey very dry, with the goal that the herb spread sticks better. Rub the spread everywhere throughout the top and sides of the turkey bosom. (It's alright in the event that it doesn't completely spread, simply pat it down admirably well.)

3. Grease the base of the slow cooker with more spread. Spot the onion inside and pour the chicken stock over it. Put the turkey bosom on the onion.

4. Cover the pot and cook it for 6-8 hours on low or 4-5 hours on high, until the inner temperature comes to at any rate 160 degrees F (71 degrees C) inside (it will rise another 5 degrees during searing and resting). On the off chance that you can, lift the cover about an hour into cooking and utilize a baked good brush to spread the herb margarine all the more uniformly absurd and sides of the turkey. (Try not to utilize dissolved margarine from the earliest starting point since it will all dribble off the without any weaning period.)

5. When the turkey is done, dispose of the onions yet spare the fluid below, which you can use as chicken soup in recipes!

6. Toward the end, preheat the oven and spot the rack close to it, with simply enough space for the turkey to fit underneath. Move the turkey bosom to a preparing dish or simmering container, and cook for 4-8

minutes, until caramelized. Rest for 10 minutes before cutting.

NUTRITION INFORMATION
Calories317 | Fat17g | Protein39g | Total Carbs1g | Net Carbs1g | Fiber0g | Sugar0g

SIMMERING POT LOW CARB KETO TACO CASSEROLE RECIPE

This easy low carb keto taco meal formula has only 4 grams net carbs! Perceive how to make Crock-Pot taco meal with only 10 minutes Prep and basic ingredients - the slow Cooker accomplishes all the work.

Course Main: Course

Cooking: Mexican

Calories: 612 kcal

Prep Time: 5 minutes

Cook Time: 2 hours 15 minutes

Total Time: 2 hours 20 minutes

Serving size: 1/2 cups, or 1/6 whole formula

INGREDIENTS
Taco Casserole:
1 tbsp avocado oil
2 lb ground meat
3/4 cup water
1/4 cup taco flavouring
2 huge Bell peppers (diced; utilize orange or yellow for shading assortment)
1/4 huge Onion (diced)
2 10-oz jars diced tomatoes with green chiles (depleted quite well - push down while depleting; see note on less hot alternative*)
1 cup cheddar

Discretionary Toppings:
Iceberg lettuce (destroyed)
Fresh tomatoes (diced)
Avocados (cubed)
Fresh cilantro (cleaved)
Sour cream

DIRECTIONS

1. In a huge saute dish, heat avocado oil over medium-high warmth. Include the ground hamburger. Cook, breaking separated with a spatula, for 8-10 minutes, until seared.

2. Add the water and taco flavouring. Heat to the point of boiling, at that point stew for 2-5 minutes, until it thickens and taco meat structures.

3. Transfer the meat to the 7 QT Crock-Pot Cook and carry easy clean slow cooker. Include the diced peppers, onions, and depleted diced tomatoes with green chiles. Combine everything.

4. Cover the slow Cooker with the cover and Cook for 4 hours on Low or 2-3 hours on High. Now you can take your Crock-Pot Cook and Carry anyplace you have to (utilize the side hooks to seal the cover), and simply plug it in to keep it warm when you arrive.

5. Right before serving, mix the goulash. (You can spoon out any abundance fluid that may have aggregated, yet there shouldn't be a lot in the event that you depleted the tomatoes well.) Set the Crock-Pot slow Cooker to High and sprinkle destroyed cheddar on top. Spread and cook for around 5 minutes, until the cheddar softens.

6. Top your goulash with any garnishes you like, for example, lettuce, tomatoes, avocados and additionally cilantro.

* This makes a really fiery taco goulash. If you incline toward it progressively gentle, you can sub either of the jars of diced tomatoes with green chiles with plain diced tomatoes. Including harsh cream for trimming will likewise mellow it out.

NUTRITION INFORMATION
Calories612 | Fat43g | Protein48g | Total Carbs6g | Net Carbs4g | Fiber2g | Sugar2g

Nutrition data does exclude discretionary fixings, since what you include, and how much, will fluctuate.

FLAWLESS GARLIC BUTTER PRIME RIB ROAST RECIPE

A definitive manual for flawless prime rib broil! Incorporates how to cook prime rib (with cooking time per pound graph), my tasty garlic margarine prime rib formula, the amount to serve, and that's only the tip of the iceberg.

Course: Main Course

Cooking: American

Calories: 575 kcal

Prep Time: 5 minutes

Cook Time: 1 hour 15 minutes

Resting: Time 20 minutes

Total Time: 2 hours 20 minutes

Serving size: ~6.5 ounces, or around 1/20 of the whole dish

INGREDIENTS

1 4-bone Standing rib broil (~8 lbs including bones)

1 1/2 tbsp sea salt

1 tsp Black pepper

6 tbsp butter (3/4 stick, liquefied)

2 tbsp Italian flavouring

1 head garlic (minced; around 10-12 cloves or 5-6 tsp minced)

DIRECTION

1. Place the prime rib, greasy side up, onto a Cooking skillet fitted with a broiling rack. Season generously with ocean salt and dark pepper.

2. Preheat the stove to 450 degrees F (232 degrees C).

3. In a little bowl, mix together the spread, Italian flavouring, and minced garlic. Pour the blend over the prime rib and utilize a seasoning brush to spread equally.

4. Roast the prime rib in the broiler, revealed, for 20 to 30 minutes, until the garlic on top is dull brilliant dark-coloured,

yet not consumed. Tent the highest point of the prime rib with foil. Decrease stove temperature to 350 degrees F (176 degrees C) and keep broiling until the prime rib arrives at your ideal inner temperature:

* 110 F (43 C) for uncommon - roughly 55 to 65 minutes

* 115 F (46 C) for medium uncommon - roughly 60 to 70 minutes

* 125 F (51 C) for medium - roughly 65 to 80 minutes

For medium uncommon, it will take roughly an extra 8 to 9 minutes for every kg of meat after the underlying high-temp cook at 450 degrees F (232 degrees C). The above meat temperatures are not last temperatures, simply the temperature to reach in the stove. The inward temperature will rise another 20 degrees in the following stage.

5. Remove the prime rib from the broiler. Let it rest for an extra 20 minutes before cutting, to come up to the correct temperature and complete the process of Cooking.

NUTRITION INFORMATION
Calories575 | Fat51g | Protein24g | Total
Carbs0g | Net Carbs0g | Fiber0g | Sugar

EASY LOW CARB KETO BEEF STEW RECIPE

This easy keto hamburger stew formula takes only 10 minutes to prep, with a mystery fixing that suggests a flavour like potatoes. Low carb hamburger stew is rich and generous - without the carbs!

Course Main: Course

Food: American

Calories: 410 kcal

Prep Time: 10 minutes

Cook Time: 1 hour 20 minutes

Total Time: 1 hour 30 minutes

Serving size: 1 cup
INGREDIENTS
2 lb Beef toss stew meat (cut into 1-inch pieces)
1/2 tsp Sea salt
1/4 tsp Black pepper
2 tbsp Olive oil (isolated)
1 medium onion (diced)
2 medium Carrots (stripped, cut into 1/4-inch-thick-circles)
2 cloves Garlic (minced)
1 tsp Italian flavouring
1 lb Celery root (weight stripped and cubed; from ~1.5 lb with strip and stems)
6 cups Beef bone juices
1 14.5-oz can diced tomatoes
2 medium Bay leaves

DIRECTIONS

1. Season the hamburger with salt and pepper. (It will be a light sum on the grounds that the soup will be salty.)

2. Heat a tablespoon of oil in a huge dutch stove over medium warmth. Include the meat in a solitary layer. (Work in groups on

the off chance that you can't get the hamburger in a solitary layer on the base of the dish.) Sear for around 8-10 minutes Totals for every clump, moving just like clockwork after each side has very much carmelized. Expel the meat and put aside on a plate.

3. Heat another tablespoon of oil in a similar dutch stove. Include the onions and carrots. Saute for around 10 minutes, until delicate and gently sautéed.

4. Add the garlic and Italian flavouring. Saute for about a moment, until fragrant.

5. Place the meat once again into the dutch stove. Include the stock, diced tomatoes, and entire straight leaves. Scratch any caramelized bits from the base of the pot.

6. Bring the meat stew to a bubble, at that point diminish warmth to medium-low and stew for a 45-an hour, until hamburger is delicate.

7. Add the celery root—increment warmth to heat to the point of boiling once more.

Spread and stew for around 15 minutes, until delicate.

8. Remove the straight leaves. Modify salt and pepper to taste if necessary.

NUTRITION INFORMATION
Calories410 | Fat22g | Protein36g | Total Carbs14g | Net Carbs11g | Fiber3g | Sugar4g

THE BEST BROILED LOBSTER TAIL RECIPE

This guide has all you have to think about Cooking lobster tails - how to prepare lobster tails (butterfly them), how to cook lobster tails, and the best seared lobster tail formula - all in only 20 minutes!

Course: Main Course

Food: American

Calories: 337 kcal

Prep Time: 10 minutes

Cook Time: 10 minutes

Total Time: 20 minutes

Serving size: 1 10-ounce lobster tail

INGREDIENTS
4 Lobster tails (10 oz each)

1/4 cup Salted margarine (dissolved; 1/2 stick)
2 cloves garlic (Squashed)
2 tsp lemon juice
1/2 tsp smoked paprika
1 squeeze Cayenne pepper

DIRECTIONS

1.If tails are solidified, defrost them medium-term in the ice chest, or in a sack submerged in cool water on the counter for around 30 minutes.

2. Preheat the stove to Broil (500 degrees F or 260 degrees C). Flush the defrosted lobster shells. Set the stove rack to such an extent that lobster tails set on a heating sheet would be 4 to 5 inches from the oven.

3. Butterfly the lobster tails. Utilizing kitchen shears, chop down the focal point of the shell the long way, beginning from the end inverse the tail blades, proceeding down until you arrive at the tail however without cutting the tail. You need to slice through the highest point of the shell, yet don't slice through the base shell. Utilize your thumbs and fingers to spread open the shell on top, at that point delicately pull the lobster meat

upward, isolating it away from the base shell, leaving the end joined to the tail balance unblemished. Marginally push together the unfilled shell underneath and place the column of meat on top. Spot the butterflied lobster tail onto the Preparing sheet.

4. In a little bowl, whisk together the dissolved margarine, garlic, lemon juice, smoked paprika, and cayenne. Brush the spread blend over the lobster meat.

5. Broil the lobster tails until the meat is misty and daintily sautéed, around 1 moment for each ounce of the individual tail. (For instance, sear for 10-ounce lobster tails for 10 minutes.)

NUTRITION INFORMATION
Calories337 | Fat13g | Protein50g | Total Carbs0g | Net Carbs0g | Fiber0g | Sugar0g

KETO SESAME ASIAN KELP NOODLES RECIPE

This healthy, easy kelp noodles formula is brimming with delicate chicken, fresh veggies, sesame sauce, and Asian kelp noodles. Keto, paleo, and prepared shortly!

Course: Main Course

Food: Japanese

Calories: 394 kcal

Prep Time: 5 minutes

Cook Time: 22 minutes

Total Time: 27 minutes

Serving size: 1/4 of the whole formula

INGREDIENTS

Sautéed food

1 lb Chicken bosom (cut into reduced down pieces)

12 oz Kelp noodles

10 oz Mushrooms (cut)

2 cup Broccoli (cut into little florets)

3 enormous Carrots (cut into scaled-down pieces)

1 tsp Olive oil

Sauce

1/3 cup Coconut aminos

2 tbsp toasted sesame oil

2 cloves Garlic (minced or squashed)

3 tbsp Sesame seeds

DIRECTIONS

1. Heat the olive oil in a huge skillet or wok over medium warmth. Fry the mushrooms for around 5-8 minutes, until the fluid from the mushrooms, has dissipated.

2. Add the chicken pieces, carrots, and broccoli (centre around the chicken contacting the dish). Sautéed food for 6-8

minutes, until the chicken is nearly cooked through however not dry.

3.To make the sauce, whisk together the coconut aminos, toasted sesame oil, garlic, and sesame seeds.

4. Add the kelp noodles and sauce blend to the container. Sautéed food for around 5 minutes, until warmed through. Season with ocean salt to taste if necessary.

NUTRITION INFORMATION
Calories394 | Fat21g | Protein38g | Total Carbs14g | Net Carbs6g | Fiber8g | Sugar3g

RICH GARLIC CHICKEN THIGHS RECIPE

Garlic spread chicken thighs make an ideal low carb chicken dinner! This velvety garlic chicken formula is extravagant enough for visitors, however easy enough for weeknights.

Course: Main Course

Food: American, Spanish

Calories: 297 kcal

Prep Time: 5 minutes

Cook Time: 20 minutes

Total Time: 25 minutes

Servings

INGREDIENTS
1 1/3 lb of boneless skinless chicken thighs(~8 medium)
1/2 tsp Sea salt

1/4 tsp smoked paprika

1/8 tsp Black pepper

2 tbsp butter (isolated)

1/2 head garlic (stripped and cut meagerly; 6 cloves)

1/2 cup chicken bone juices (or normal chicken soup)

1/2 cup white cooking wine

1/4 cup Heavy cream

1 medium Bay leaf

DIRECTIONS

1. Season the chicken on the two sides with the salt, pepper, and smoked paprika.

2. Heat 1 tablespoon (30 grams) spread in an enormous skillet or saute a dish, over medium-high warmth. Include the chicken and burn for 5 to 7 minutes for every side, without moving, until caramelized and cooked.

3. Remove the chicken from the dish, spread with foil and put in a safe spot.

4. Add the rest of the tablespoon (30 grams) margarine to the skillet. Include the cut garlic. Saute for 2-3 minutes, frequently

blending, until the garlic is fragrant and beginning to dark-coloured.

5. Add the stock and wine to the container. Utilize a wooden spoon to scratch any sautéed bits from the base (this is called de-coating).

6. Place the sound leaf into the container and submerge. Carry the fluid to a delicate bubble, at that point decrease warmth and stew for 8-12 minutes, until the volume is diminished considerably.

7. Add the cream to the container—warmth for only a couple of moments (don't bubble).

8. Remove the cove leaf and add the chicken back to the container. Spoon the sauce over the chicken.

NUTRITION INFORMATION
Calories297 | Fat17g | Protein30g | Total Carbs1g | Net Carbs1g | Fiber0g | Sugar0g

KETO GROUND BEEF CAULIFLOWER LASAGNA RECIPE

Perceive how to make keto lasagna with cauliflower! This cauliflower lasagna formula is made with cauliflower lasagna noodles, layers of ground meat marinara, and gooey cheddar.

Course: Main Course

Cooking: Italian

Calories: 386 kcal

Prep Time: 10 minutes

Cook Time: 30 minutes

Total Time: 40 minutes

Serving size: 1 cup

INGREDIENTS
1 head Cauliflower (cut into florets)

1 tbsp Olive oil
1 lb ground meat
1/2 huge Onion (slashed)
2 cloves Garlic (minced)
1 cup Marinara sauce
1 (14.5 oz) can diced tomatoes
1/2 cup Fresh basil (slashed, partitioned)
1 cup Mozzarella cheddar (destroyed)
Sea salt
Black pepper

DIRECTIONS

1. Preheat the broiler to 400 degrees F (204 degrees C). Softly oil a cycle 9 in (23 cm) or square 9x9 in (23x23 cm) goulash dish (line with foil whenever wanted).

2. Toss the cauliflower with olive oil. Sprinkle softly with ocean salt and dark pepper. Broil for 15-20 minutes, mixing part of the way through, until fresh delicate.

3. Cook the onion or 8-10 min. over the medium-low warmth, until translucent and somewhat seared.

4. Add the ground meat—increment warmth to medium-high. Cook for around 8-10

minutes, breaking separated with a spatula until seared.

5. Stir the garlic together, marinara sauce, diced tomatoes, and half of the new basil—season with ocean salt and dark pepper to taste. Cook for 2 minutes, until warmed.

6. Pour the tomato meat sauce over the cauliflower. Sprinkle with destroyed mozzarella cheddar. Prepare for 8-10 minutes, until the cheddar bubbles. Top with the staying new basil strips.

NUTRITION INFORMATION
Calories386 | Fat24g | Protein28g | Total Carbs13g | Net Carbs10g | Fiber3g | Sugar6g

*Nutrition information will differ marginally relying on upon the brand of marinara sauce.

RECIPES FOR DESSERTS

LOW CARB KETO HOT CHOCOLATE RECIPE

Perceive how to make keto hot cocoa with only 5 ingredients! This without sugar low carb hot cocoa formula is thick and rich, yet easy. Conjecture the mystery element for the best keto hot cocoa ever!

Course: Dessert, Drinks

Cooking: French

Calories: 193 kcal

Prep Time: 5 minutes

Cook Time: 5 minutes

Total Time: 10 minutes

Serving size: 1 coffee size mug, or 1/4 of the whole formula

INGREDIENTS

6 oz High-quality dim chocolate (cleaved or chocolate chips; use without sugar whenever wanted)

1/2 cup unsweetened almond milk (or customary milk)

1/2 cup Heavy cream (or coconut cream for paleo)

1 tbsp Allulose (can preclude or utilize any sugar of decision)

1/2 tsp Vanilla concentrate

DIRECTIONS

1. Heat almond milk, cream, and sugar in a little pot over medium warmth until it stews tenderly. Expel from heat.

2. Stir in vanilla concentrate and chocolate. Whisk continually until liquefied. Fill coffee cups to serve.

NUTRITION INFORMATION

Calories193 | Fat18g | Protein2g | Total Carbs4g | Net Carbs1g | Fiber3g | Sugar0.1g

*Nutrition information may fluctuate contingent upon which chocolate bar you

use. Use sans sugar chocolate, not unsweetened

LOW CARB KETO SNICKERDOODLES COOKIE RECIPE

This keto snickerdoodle treat formula lets you appreciate a treat exemplary with just 3g net carbs! Perceive how to make low carb snickerdoodles in only 30 minutes.

Course: Dessert

Food: American

Calories: 193 kcal

Prep Time: 15 minutes

Cook Time: 15 minutes

Total Time: 30 minutes

Serving size: 1 treat

INGREDIENTS

Cookies:

6 tbsp Salted margarine

1/3 cup Golden priest organic product sugar mix

1/2 tbsp Cinnamon

1/2 tsp Xanthan gum

1/2 tsp sans gluten heating powder

1 enormous Egg

1 tsp Vanilla concentrate

2 1/2 cups Blanched almond flour

Covering:

1 1/2 tbsp Golden priest organic product sugar mix

1 1/2 tsp Cinnamon

DIRECTIONS

1. Preheat the broiler to 350 degrees F (177 degrees C). Line a heating sheet with material paper.

2. Using a hand blender at medium speed, cream margarine, and sugar together until fleecy.

3. Beat in the cinnamon, thickener, and Preparing powder. Beat in the egg and vanilla concentrate.

5. In a different little bowl, mix together the sugar mix and cinnamon for the covering.

6. Use a medium treat scoop to scoop the mixture and press into the scoop. Discharge and fold into a ball. Roll the ball in the cinnamon covering. Spot onto the lined Preparing sheet and straighten utilizing your palm. Rehash with outstanding treat mixture, putting the cookies in any event 1.5 inches (4 cm) separated in the wake of levelling.

7. Bake for 15-20 min., until brilliant. Cool Totally before moving.

NUTRITION INFORMATION
Calories193 | Fat17g | Protein5g | Total Carbs5g | Net Carbs3g | Fiber2g Sugar0g

ALMOND FLOUR KETO SHORTBREAD COOKIES RECIPE

this rich keto shortbread cookies formula with almond flour has only 4 ingredients and 1g net carb each! low carb almond flour cookies taste simply like genuine shortbread. nobody can tell they're sans gluten shortbread cookies.

Course: Dessert

Cooking: American

Calories: 124 kcal

Prep Time: 10 minutes

Cook Time: 12 minutes

Total Time: 22 minutes

Serving size: 1 treat

INGREDIENTS
Basic Keto Shortbread Cookies
2 1/2 cups Blanched almond flour
6 tbsp Butter (mellowed; can utilize coconut oil for without dairy, yet flavour and surface will be extraordinary)
1/2 cup unadulterated allulose or unadulterated erythritol
1 tsp Vanilla concentrate

Discretionary Chocolate Dip
1/2 cup sans sugar chocolate chips
2 tsp Coconut oil
3 tbsp Pecans (slashed)

DIRECTIONS
Basic Keto Shortbread Cookies
1. Preheat the broiler to 350 degrees F (177 degrees C). Line a treat sheet with material paper.

2. Use a hand blender or stand blender to beat together the margarine and erythritol, until it's cushy and light in shading.

3. Beat in the vanilla concentrate. The batter will be thick and somewhat brittle, however, should stick when squeezed together.)

4. Scoop adjusted tablespoonfuls of the mixture onto the prepared treat sheet. Smooth every treat to around 1/3 in (.8 cm) thick. Remember they won't extend or far-out during heating, so make them as dainty as you need them when done.)

5. Allow cooling totally in the dish before dealing with (Cookies will solidify as they cool).

Discretionary Chocolate Dip
1. Allow without gluten shortbread cookies to cool and solidify totally before plunging in chocolate.

2. Melt without sugar chocolate and coconut oil in a twofold heater. When liquefied, plunge the cookies most of the way into the chocolate and spot onto the lined dish. Promptly sprinkle with hacked nuts before the chocolate sets.

3. Chill in the cooler before taking care of, until the chocolate is firm.

*Nutrition information does exclude discretionary chocolate plunge and walnuts.

*The salted spread is suggested. In the case of utilizing unsalted, include couple portions of ocean salt to the mixture in stage 3.

NUTRITION INFORMATION
Calories124 | Fat12g | Protein3g | Total Carbs3.3g | Net Carbs1.7g | Fiber1.6g| Sugar1g

LOW CARB PALEO KETO BLUEBERRY MUFFINS RECIPE WITH ALMOND FLOUR

Perceive how to make the best keto biscuits in only 30 minutes! These ultra-soggy almond flour blueberry biscuits without any Preparation are speedy and easy. It's the ideal low carb paleo blueberry biscuits formula - and the just a single you'll ever require.

Course: Breakfast, Snack

Food: American

Calories: 217 kcal
 Prep Time: 10 minutes

Cook Time: 20 minutes

Total Time: 30 minutes

Serving size: 1 biscuit

 INGREDIENTS
2 1/2 cup Blanched almond flour
1/2 cup Erythritol (or any granulated sugar)
1 1/2 tsp sans gluten Preparing powder
1/4 tsp Sea salt (discretionary, however, suggested)
1/3 cup Coconut oil (estimated strong, at that point liquefied; can likewise utilize spread)
1/3 cup unsweetened almond milk
3 huge Eggs
1/2 tsp Vanilla concentrate
3/4 cup Blueberries

DIRECTIONS

1. Prc-heat the stove to 350 degrees F (177 degrees C). Line a biscuit skillet with 10 or 12 silicone or material paper biscuit liners. (Utilize 12 for lower calories/carbs, or 10 for bigger biscuit tops.)

2. In an enormous bowl, mix together the almond flour, erythritol, preparing powder and ocean salt.

3. Mix in the softened coconut oil, almond milk, eggs, and vanilla concentrate. Overlay in the blueberries.

4. Distribute the player equally among the biscuit cups. Heat for around 20-25 minutes, until the top is brilliant and an embedded toothpick tells the truth.

NUTRITION INFORMATION

Calories217 | Fat19g | Protein7g | Total Carbs6g | Net Carbs3g | Fiber3g | Sugar2g

KETO PIÑA COLADA CHEESECAKE CUPCAKES RECIPE

This piña cheesecake cupcakes formula resembles keto smaller than usual cheesecake with pineapple and coconut enhance! It just takes 25 minutes to make these pineapple keto cheesecake cupcakes.

Course: Dessert

Food: American

Calories: 246 kcal

Prep Time: 10 minutes

Cook Time: 15 minutes

Total Time: 25 minutes

Serving size: 1 cupcake

INGREDIENTS

Pineapple chccsecake filling

16 oz Cream cheddar (relaxed at room temperature)

1 8-oz can Pineapple lumps (depleted well)

1 enormous Egg (beaten)

1/2 cup Powdered erythritol

2 tsp Vanilla concentrate

1/2 tsp Coconut separate (discretionary, on the off chance that you need coconut to enhance in the filling)

Shortbread outside layer

3/4 cup Coconut flour

1/4 cup Coconut oil (softened)

2 enormous Egg (beaten)

1 tbsp Erythritol (or any sugar of decision)

1 squeeze Sea salt

Beating

1/4 cup Coconut drops (unsweetened)

DIRECTIONS

1. Preheat the broiler to 350 degrees F (177 degrees C). Line a biscuit tin with silicone or material paper cupcake liners.

2. In an enormous bowl, combine the outside layer ingredients until brittle. Press

the outside layer into the bottoms of the cupcake liners. Put in a safe spot.

3. Spoon the filling equitably on the cupcake outside layers. Sprinkle coconut drops on top.

4. Bake for 13-17 minutes, until the coconut drops begin to turn brilliant however the inside is still jiggly. Cool totally, at that point refrigerate for at any rate 30 minutes, or until set, before serving. Serve beat with natively constructed whipped cream.

NUTRITION INFORMATION
Calories246 | Fat22g | Protein7g | Total Carbs10g | Net Carbs5g | Fiber5g | Sugar4g

KETO FRENCH ALMOND CAKE RECIPE

Perceive how to make keto almond flour cake with 4g net carbs! This easy toasted almond cake formula is flavorful and suggests a flavour like a genuine French almond cake.

Course: Dessert

Food: French

Calories: 339 kcal

Prep Time: 15 minutes

Cook Time: 35 minutes

Total Time: 50 minutes

Serving size: 1 cut, or 1/12 whole formula

INGREDIENTS

Cake:
3 1/2 cups Blanched almond flour
1/2 tbsp sans gluten preparing powder
1/4 tsp Sea salt
1/3 cup Butter (relaxed)
1/2 cup of besti monk fruit erythritol blend
4 big Eggs
3/4 cup sour cream
1/2 tsp Vanilla concentrate
1/2 tsp almond separate

Coating:
3 tbsp Butter (dissolved)
1/4 tsp Almond extricate
1/4 tsp Vanilla concentrate

Toasted almonds:
1/2 cup sliced almonds

DIRECTIONS

1. Preheat the stove at 350 degrees F (177 degrees C). Line the base of a springform skillet or cake dish with material paper.

2. Arrange almonds in a solitary layer on a Preparing sheet. Toast for 3-4 minutes, until brilliant. Expel from the broiler and allow to cool. Leave the stove on.

3. Meanwhile, bcat spread and sugar together.

4. Beat in almond flour, Preparing powder, and ocean salt.

5. Beat in eggs, sharp cream, vanilla and almond separate.

6. Bake at (177 degrees C) for 28-32 minutes, until the top is brilliant and springs back, and embedded toothpick tells the truth.

7. Allow the cake to cool for in any event 10 minutes in the skillet, until warm yet no longer hot.

8. Meanwhile, whisk together the coating ingredients.

9. On the off chance that you utilized a springform container, discharge and expelled the sides (you can keep it sitting on the base part). In the event that you utilized a cake container, cautiously flip over a towel, at that point flip again with the goal that the cake is straight up.

10. Place the cake onto a wire rack. While the cake is still warm, utilize a baked good brush to brush the coating over the cake, saving 1 tablespoon (14 ml) of the coating.

11. Sprinkle the rest of the tablespoon of coating on the almonds to help seal them.

12. Let the cake cool totally. Whenever wanted, sprinkle with increasingly powdered sugar for serving.

NUTRITION INFORMATION
Calories339 | Fat31g | Protein10g | Total Carbs8g | Net Carbs4g | Fiber4g | Sugar1g

THE LOW-CARB KETO CHOCOLATE CHIP COOKIES RECIPE WITH ALMOND FLOUR

The best keto chocolate chip cookies ever! This sans sugar low carb chocolate chip Cookies formula needs just 6 ingredients and 10 minutes Prep.

Course: Dessert

Cooking: American

Calories: 140 kcal

Prep Time: 10 minutes

Cook Time: 12 minutes

Total Time: 22 minutes

Serving size: 1 treat

INGREDIENTS

2 1/2 cup Blanched almond flour

1/2 cup Butter (mollified; can utilize coconut oil for without dairy, yet flavour and surface will be extraordinary) *

1 huge Egg

1/2 cup Allulose (suggested for delicate Cookies, yet erythritol will work for crisper ones)

1 tsp Vanilla concentrate

1 tsp Blackstrap molasses (discretionary, yet suggested for best flavour)

1/2 tsp Xanthan gum (discretionary, yet suggested for best surface)

1/2 cup without sugar dull chocolate chips

*Salted spread is prescribed. In the case of utilizing unsalted, include couple portions of ocean salt to the batter in stage 3.

DIRECTIONS

1. Pre-heat to 350 degrees F (177 degrees C). Line a treat sheet with material paper.

2. Use a hand blender or stand blender to beat together the spread and erythritol, until it's cushy and light in shading.

3. Beat in the egg, vanilla concentrate, and blackstrap molasses, if utilizing.

4. If utilizing thickener, sprinkles (don't dump) it over the treat batter, at that point beat in utilizing the hand blender.

5. Fold in the chocolate chips.

6. Use a medium treat scoop to drop adjusted tablespoonfuls of the batter onto the Prepared treat sheet. Level every treat to around 1/3 in (.8 cm) thick. Remember they just spread a little and don't far out during heating, so make them as slender as you need them when done.

7. Bake for 12 min., until the edges are brilliant. (Time will fluctuate dependent on your broiler and thickness of your cookies.) Allow cooling totally in the dish before taking care of.

NUTRITION INFORMATION
Calories140 | Fat13g | Protein4g | Total Carbs5g | Net Carbs2g | Fiber3g | Sugar1g

SUGAR-FREF KETO CHOCOLATE FROSTING RECIPE

Perceive how to make without sugar keto chocolate icing that poses a flavour like the genuine article! My easy keto low carb keto icing formula takes only 5 ingredients + 5 minutes.

Course: Dessert

Food: American

Calories: 131 kcal

Cook Time: 5 minutes

Total Time: 5 minutes

Serving size: 2 tablespoons

INGREDIENTS
1 1/2 cups Butter (mollified)
10 tbsp of cocoa powder (1/2 cup + 2 tbsp)

1/2 cup Powdered Monk Fruit
Allulose Blend
1 tsp Vanilla concentrate
1 tbsp Heavy cream

DIRECTIONS

1. Using a hand blender in a bowl, beat the spread for around 1 moment, until cushy.

2. Sugar, and vanilla concentrate, beginning at low speed and expanding to high once it gets fused. Beat for 30 seconds on high.

3. Beat in overwhelming cream. (You can add more to disperse varying.) Start low, at that point beat for 30 seconds on high once more, until smooth and cushy.

NUTRITION INFORMATION

Calories131 | Fat14g | Protein1g | Total Carbs2g | Net Carbs1g | Fiber1g | Sugar1g

LOW CARB-KETO CHOCOLATE & CUPCAKES RECIPE

Perceive how to make keto chocolate cupcakes with almond flour and no sugar! This keto low carb chocolate cupcakes formula is rich, sweet, and prepared in a short time.

Course: Dessert

Food: American

Calories: 479 kcal

Prep Time: 10 minutes

Cook Time: 20 minutes

Total Time: 30 minutes

Serving size: 1 keto cupcake

INGREDIENTS
2 cups Blanched almond flour
6 tbsp Cocoa powder

1/2 tbsp sans gluten heating powder
1/4 tsp Sea salt
1/3 cup Butter (mellowed)
 1/2 cup of Monk Fruit Erythritol Blend (or 2/3 cup on the off chance that you have a solid sweet tooth)
3 enormous Eggs
1/2 cup unsweetened almond milk
1 tsp Vanilla concentrate
1/2 formula Keto Chocolate Frosting (1/4 cups)

DIRECTIONS
1. Preheat the broiler to 350 degrees F (176 degrees C). Line 10 cups in a biscuit tin with paper liners.

2. In an enormous bowl, utilize a hand blender to beat spread and sugar together, until cushy.

3. Beat in almond flour, cocoa powder, heating powder, and ocean salt.

4. Beat in eggs, almond milk, and vanilla concentrate.

5. Bake for 20-25 minutes, until a toothpick embedded in the focal point of a cupcake, confesses all.

6. Allow biscuits to cool totally, at that point ice with keto chocolate icing (around 2 tablespoons icing for each cupcake).

This low carb formula was highlighted in the February 2020 Keto Cooking Challenge!

NUTRITION INFORMATION
Calories479 | Fat48g | Protein10g | Total Carbs11g | Net Carbs6g | Fiber5g | Sugar3g

LOW CARB-KETO CREAM CHEESE FROSTING WITHOUT POWDERED SUGAR

Need to perceive how to make cream cheddar icing without powdered sugar? It's so easy! This delightful, low carb keto cream cheddar icing formula has only 5 ingredients. Use without sugar keto cream cheddar icing to ice cupcakes, cakes, and that's just the beginning.

Course: Dessert

Food: American

Calories: 110 kcal

Prep Time: 5 minutes

Total Time: 5 minutes

Serving size: 2 tbsp

INGREDIENTS

4 oz Cream cheddar (relaxed, cut into 3D shapes)

2 tbsp Butter (relaxed, cut into 3D shapes)

1/2 cup of powdered allulose (or powdered erythritol)

1 tsp of vanilla concentrate

1 tbsp Heavy cream (or more if necessary)

DIRECTIONS

1. Use a hand blender to beat together the cream cheddar and margarine, until cushioned.

2. Beat vanilla, until very much fused.

3. Add cream and beat once more, until velvety. You can change the measure of cream to wanted consistency.

NUTRITION INFORMATION

Calories110 | Fat11g | Protein1g | Total Carbs1g | Net Carbs1g | Fiber0g | Sugar0.1g

COCONUT FLOUR KETO SUGAR COOKIES RECIPE

Low carb keto sugar cookies with coconut flour are ideal for any occasion! This 20-minute keto sugar treat formula has without sugar choices for sprinkles and icing, as well.

Course: Dessert

Cooking: American

Calories: 61 kcal

Prep Time: 12 minutes

Cook Time: 8 minutes

Total Time: 20 minutes

Serving size: 1 little treat

INGREDIENTS
Coconut Flour Sugar Cookies:
1/3 cup Butter (mellowed, or coconut oil for without dairy)
1/3 cup Allulose

2 huge Eggs
1/2 tsp Vanilla concentrate
1/2 tsp Baking powder
1/4 tsp Sea salt
1/2 cup Coconut flour
1/4 tsp Xanthan gum (discretionary, for milder, sturdier, and less brittle cookies)

Discretionary Toppings:
2/3 formula Keto Cream Cheese Frosting
4 tsp without sugar sprinkles

DIRECTIONS
1. Preheat the stove to 350 degrees F (176 degrees C). Line a preparing sheet with material paper.

2. In a profound bowl, utilize a hand blender to beat together the spread and sugar, until cushy.

3. Beat in the eggs, vanilla, heating powder, and ocean salt.

4. Gradually beat in the coconut flour.

5. Sprinkle (don't dump) the thickener over the treat mixture, at that point beat in. Let

the treat batter sit for a couple of moments to thicken.

6. Baking alternative 1: utilize a little treat scoop to scoop the batter onto the Preparing sheet. Smooth with your palm to 1/4 inch thick (they won't spread much during heating), keeping them at any rate an inch separated.

Preparing choice 2: structure the batter into a ball and chill for 60 minutes. When the treat mixture is firm, expel it from the cooler and spot between two bits of material paper. Turn out to around 1/4-inch thick. Cut into shapes utilizing dough shapers. You can expel the abundance batter away from the patterns and simply leave the cookies on the material paper, at that point, slide onto the heating sheet. Then again, you can cautiously utilize a slim turner to move the pattern cookies to the material lined heating sheet. Any treat batter you tore away from the pattern, you can shape a ball with it and turn out again to make more cookies.

7. Bake for around 7-8 minutes, until Cookies begin to solidify, yet are still delicate. (They won't obscure a lot, and don't

solidify completely until after they cool.) Remove from the stove and cool totally before moving or including icing.

8. If you need cookies with icing and sprinkles, make the cream cheddar icing formula as indicated by the directions here. You'll utilize 2/3 of the whole group for the Cookies. Spread the icing over the cookies (about 1.5 tsp (7.5 g) per treat) and top with sprinkles (around 1/4 tsp (1.25 g) per treat).

NUTRITION INFORMATION
Calories61 | Fat5g | Protein1g | Total Carbs2g | Net Carbs1g | Fiber1g | Sugar1g

KETO LOW CARB PROTEIN BARS RECIPE

Crush your chocolate yearnings with this low carb keto protein bars formula in a fantastic chocolate hazelnut enhance! These high protein low carb bars have quite recently 2g net carbs + 8g protein.

Course: Snack

Cooking: American

Calories: 182 kcal

Prep Time: 15 minutes

Total Time: 15 minutes

Serving size: 1 bar, or 1/12 of the formula

INGREDIENTS
1 1/4 cups Blanched hazelnuts (separated into 1 cup and 1/4 cup)
1 cup Blanched almond flour
2 tbsp Cocoa powder
1/4 cup Collagen protein powder

1/2 cup besti powdered priest natural product allulose mix
1/4 tsp Sea salt
2 tbsp Almond spread (the somewhat runny kind)
1 oz Cocoa spread (dissolved)
Without sugar chocolate chips (dissolved; discretionary, for sprinkling)

DIRECTIONS
1. Line an 8x8 container with material paper, allowing it to hang over at any rate 2 sides.

2. Place 1 cup (120 g) hazelnuts into a food processor. Heartbeat until you get a fine meal-like consistency.

3. Add the almond flour, cocoa powder, protein powder, Besti, and ocean salt. Heartbeat a couple of times, just until blended. Scratch the sides of the food processor and heartbeat once more.

4. Add the almond spread and liquefied cocoa margarine. Procedure constantly until a batter structures, pulls from the inside, feels firm to the touch, and leaves a unique mark when squeezed. It ought to be firm and

sparkly, not runny or brittle. In the event that it's not uniform, you may need to physically mix and scratch the sides, at that point procedure more.

5. Press the protein bar mixture firmly and uniformly into the lined skillet. Hack the staying 1/4 cup (30 g) hazelnuts and press into the top. Whenever wanted, shower with liquefied chocolate (discretionary).

6. Place the skillet in the ice chest and chill for at any rate 1-2 hours, or until exceptionally firm. Lift the bars out of the dish utilizing the edges of the material paper, and cut into 12 bars, utilizing an enormous gourmet expert's blade with a straight down movement or shaking movement (don't see-saw, or bars may disintegrate).

7. Store bars in the cooler, between layers of material paper.

NUTRITION INFORMATION
Calories182 | Fat16g | Protein8g Total Carbs5g | Net Carbs2g | Fiber3g | Sugar1g

LOW CARB PALEO-KETO RECIPE & CHOCOLATE MUG

Perceive how to make a keto mug cake in a short time, utilizing 6 ingredients! This rich, wet, low carb paleo chocolate mug cake formula has just 4 grams net carbs.

Course: Dessert

Food: American

Calories: 433 kcal

Prep Time: 2 minutes

Cook Time: 2 minutes

Total Time: 4 minutes

Serving size: 1 mug cake (whole formula)

INGREDIENTS
1 tbsp Butter (salted; *see notes for sans dairy alternatives)
3/4 oz Unsweetened heating chocolate
3 tbsp of blanched almond flour

1 1/2 tbsp of besti Monk Fruit Allulose Blend (or any granulated sugar; *see notes for choices)
1/2 tsp sans gluten Preparing powder
1 enormous Egg
1/4 tsp Vanilla concentrate (discretionary)

DIRECTIONS
Microwave Instructions
1. Melt the margarine & chocolate together in a mug or huge 12 oz (355 mL) ramekin in the microwave (around 45-60 seconds, blending part of the way through). Be mindful so as not to consume it. Ensure the ramekin is at any rate twofold the volume of the ingredients, in light of the fact that the mug cake will rise.

2. Add the almond flour, sugar, heating powder, egg, and vanilla (if utilizing). Mix everything admirably until totally combined.

3. Microwave for around 60-75 seconds, until simply firm. (Try not to over cook, or it will be dry.)

4. Serve the whipped cream, as well as sprinkle with increasingly liquefied chocolate blended with sugar.

Stove Instructions

1. Pre-heat to 350 degrees F

2. Melt the spread and chocolate together in a twofold heater on the stove. Be mindful so as not to consume it. Expel from heat.

3. Add the almond flour, sugar, preparing powder, egg, and vanilla (if utilizing). Mix everything great until totally combined.

4. Transfer the player to an enormous 12 oz (355 mL) broiler-safe ramekin (or two littler 6 oz (178 mL) ones). Ensure the ramekins are at any rate twofold the volume of the ingredients, in light of the fact that the cake will rise. Heat for around 15 minutes, until simply firm.

5. Serve the whipped cream (or potentially sprinkle with increasingly softened chocolate blended with sugar.

• For a sans dairy or paleo rendition, use ghee or coconut oil, and include a spot of salt.

• The unique variant of this formula utilized erythritol; however, the priest organic product allulose mix makes a far prevalent, very clammy mug cake. Paleo followers may like to utilize coconut sugar for the sugar.

NUTRITION INFORMATION
Calories433 | Fat38g | Protein14g | Total Carbs11g | Net Carbs4g | Fiber7g | Sugar1g

THE BEST CHAFFLES RECIPE - 5 WAYS!

All the insider facts of how to make chaffles impeccably! Incorporates the best basic keto chaffles formula, sweet chaffles (cinnamon churro + pumpkin), appetizing chaffles (jalapeno popper + garlic parmesan), tips, stunts, stunts, and substitutions.

Course: Dessert, Main Course

Cooking: American

Calories: 208 kcal

Prep Time: 5 minutes

Cook Time: 3 minutes

Total Time: 8 minutes

Serving size: 1 smaller than normal chaffle

INGREDIENTS
Basic Chaffle Recipe For Sandwiches:
1/2 cup Mozzarella cheddar (destroyed)
1 big egg
2 tbsp of blanched almond flour (or 2 tsp coconut flour)

1/2 tsp Psyllium husk powder (discretionary, yet prescribed for surface, sprinkle in, so it doesn't get bunch)
1/4 tsp Baking powder (discretionary)

Garlic Parmesan Chaffles:
1/2 cup Mozzarella cheddar (destroyed)
1/3 cup Grated Parmesan cheddar
1 huge Egg
1 clove Garlic (minced; or utilize 1/2 clove for milder garlic season)
1/2 tsp Italian flavouring
1/4 tsp Baking powder (discretionary)

Cinnamon Sugar (Churro) Chaffles:
1 huge Egg
3/4 cup Mozzarella cheddar (destroyed)
2 tbsp of blanched almond flour
1/2 tbsp Butter (dissolved)
2 tbsp Erythritol
1/2 tsp Cinnamon
1/2 tsp Vanilla concentrate
1/2 tsp Psyllium husk powder (discretionary, for surface)
1/4 tsp Baking powder (discretionary)
1 tbsp Butter (dissolved; for garnish)
1/4 cup Erythritol (for fixing)
3/4 tsp Cinnamon (for fixing)

Pumpkin Chaffles:
1/2 oz cream cheddar
1 huge egg
1/2 cup Mozzarella cheddar (destroyed)
2 tbsp pumpkin puree
2 1/2 tbsp Erythritol
3 tsp coconut flour
1/2 tbsp Pumpkin pie flavour
1/2 tsp vanilla concentrate (discretionary)
1/4 tsp baking powder (discretionary)

Zesty Jalapeno Popper Chaffles:
1 oz cream cheddar
1 enormous egg
1 cup cheddar (destroyed)
2 tbsp bacon bits
1/2 tbsp Jalapenos
1/4 tsp Baking powder (discretionary)

DIRECTIONS
1. Preheat your waffle iron for around 5 minutes, until hot.

2. If the formula contains cream cheddar, place it into a bowl first. Warmth delicately in the microwave (~15-30 seconds) or a twofold kettle, until it's delicate and easy to mix.

3. Stir in all other residual ingredients (with the exception of fixings, assuming any).

4. Pour enough of the chaffle player into the waffle creator to cover the surface well. (That is around 1/2 cup hitter for a customary waffle creator and 1/4 cup for a small scale waffle producer.)

5. Cook until caramelized and firm.

6. Carefully expel the chaffle from the waffle creator and put aside to fresh up additional. (Cooling is significant for surface!) Repeat with residual hitter, assuming any.

Unique guidance for churro chaffles as it were:
1. Stir together the erythritol and cinnamon for garnish. After the chaffles were cooked brush them with dissolved spread, at that point sprinkle done with the cinnamon "sugar" garnish (or plunge into the fixing).

The serving size of 1 smaller than normal chaffle is only for easy scaling, however, sometimes you could have two, for example, for a sandwich or full meal. The basic chaffle and garlic Parmesan recipes make 2 smaller than normal chaffles each. The cinnamon sugar (churro), pumpkin, and fiery jalapeno popper recipes make 3 small scale chaffles each. The nutrition data on the formula card is for the basic chaffles, yet you can discover nutrition information for the others in the post above.

NUTRITION INFORMATION
Calories208 | Fat16g | Protein11g | Total Carbs4g | Net Carbs2g | Fiber2g | Sugar0g

LOW CARB KETO PUMPKIN COOKIES RECIPE

This chewy, delicate keto pumpkin cookies formula makes the ideal fall dessert! Perceive how to make healthy low carb pumpkin cookies with straightforward ingredients and under 30 minutes.

Course: Dessert

Cooking: American

Calories: 110 kcal

Prep Time: 15 minutes

Cook Time: 15 minutes

Total Time: 30 minutes

Serving size: 1 2-inch treat

INGREDIENTS
Pumpkin Cookies
1/4 cup of butter (unsalted)
1/3 cup of Besti Powdered Monk Fruit Erythritol Blend

1/2 cup of pumpkin puree
1 big Egg
1 tsp of Vanilla concentrate
3 cups of blanched almond flour
2 tsp of cinnamon
1/2 tsp of nutmeg
1/2 tsp without gluten heating powder
 1/4 tsp Sea salt

Discretionary:
1/4 cup of besti Powdered Monk Fruit Erythritol Blend
1/4 cup of heavy cream
1/4 tsp Vanilla

DIRECTIONS
1. Preheat the stove to 350 degrees F (176 degrees C). Line an enormous preparing sheet with material paper.

2. In a huge profound bowl, beat together the margarine and sugar, until cushioned.

3. Beat the pumpkin puree, the egg, and vanilla.

4. Beat in the almond flour, cinnamon, nutmeg, preparing powder, and ocean salt, until a uniform treat mixture structures.

5. Use a medium treat scoop to scoop wads of the mixture and pack the batter into it. Discharge onto the lined heating sheet, 2 inches (5.08 cm) separated. Utilize your palm, or the base of a glass with a winding movement, to smooth cookies to around 1/4 inch (.64 cm) thick.

6. Bake for 15 to 20 minutes, until brilliant.

7. Meanwhile, make the coating/icing, if utilizing. In a little bowl, whisk together the coating ingredients, until smooth. If that it's excessively thick, include more cream, a teaspoon at once, until it's a spreadable consistency.

8. Cool totally to solidify before moving from the skillet.

NUTRITION INFORMATION
Calories110 | Fat9g | Protein3g | Total Carbs4g | Net Carbs3g | Fiber1g | Sugar0g

ATKINS DIET FOR BEGINNERS 2021:

THE ULTIMATE GUIDE TO LIVING A LOW-CARB LIFESTYLE.

THE BIBLE OF RECIPES ON ATKINS DIET.
(IN 20 MINUTES OR LESS)

AUTHOR:

CHARLOTTE CONLAN

This document is geared towards providing exact and reliable information with regards to the topic and issue covered. The publication is sold with the idea that the publisher is not required to render accounting, officially permitted, or otherwise, qualified services. If advice is necessary, legal or professional, a practiced individual in the profession should be ordered.

From a Declaration of Principles which was accepted and approved equally by a Committee of the American Bar Association and a Committee of Publishers and Associations.

In no way is it legal to reproduce, duplicate, or transmit any part of this document in either electronic means or in printed format. Recording of this publication is strictly prohibited and any storage of this document is not allowed unless with written permission from the publisher. All rights reserved.

The information provided herein is stated to be truthful and consistent, in that any liability, in terms of inattention or otherwise, by any usage or abuse of any policies, processes, or directions contained within is the solitary and utter responsibility of the recipient reader. Under no circumstances will any legal responsibility or blame be held against the publisher for any reparation, damages, or monetary loss due to the information herein, either directly or indirectly.

Respective authors own all copyrights not held by the publisher.

The information herein is offered for informational purposes solely, and is universal as so. The presentation of the information is without contract or any type of guarantee assurance.

The trademarks that are used are without any consent, and the publication of the trademark is without permission or backing by the trademark owner. All trademarks and brands within this book are for clarifying purposes only and are owned by the owners themselves, not affiliated with this document.

TABLE OF CONTENTS

LOW CARB BREAKFAST RECIPES114

THE ATKINS DIET
BRIEF HISTORY

The founder and father of low-carb diets, Robert Atkins may not have been the first to harness the appeal of carb-free, but he was certainly the first to bring the concept to the mainstream dieting public.

In 1963, American physician and cardiologist Robert Atkins came across a study published by Dr. Alfred W. Pennington. His research explored the theory that cutting starch and sugar from the diet could lead to significant weight loss. Putting the pound-shedding theory to the test, Atkins shrunk his own bulk and adapted the findings into the diet and formidable brand we know today.

The Atkins diet is a low-carb diet, usually recommended for weight loss.

Proponents of this diet claim that you can lose weight while eating as much protein and fat as you want, as long as you avoid foods high in carbs.

Studies have shown that low-carb diets without the need of calorie counting, are effective for weight loss and can lead to various health improvements.

The Atkins diet was originally promoted by the physician Dr. Robert C. Atkins, who wrote a best-selling book about it in 1972.

Since then, the Atkins diet has been popular all over the world with many more books having been written.

The diet was originally considered unhealthy and demonized by the mainstream health authorities, mostly due to its high saturated fat content. However, new studies suggest that saturated fat is harmless. Since then, the diet has been studied thoroughly and shown to lead to greater weight loss and greater improvements in blood sugar, "good" HDL cholesterol, triglycerides and other health markers than low-fat diets.

Despite being high in fat, it does not raise "bad" LDL cholesterol on average, though this does happen in a subset of individuals.

The main reason why low-carb diets are so

effective for weight loss is that a reduction in carbs and increased protein intake lead to reduced appetite, making you eat fewer calories without having to think about it.

The Atkins diet was based on Atkins' belief that it's the carbs in our diets which are responsible for our weight gain and that by eating more protein,so we can switch on the "satiated" trigger, which helps us control our appetite. For this reason strict limits are put on carbs especially during the initial weight loss stage, but unlike most other diets there are no restrictions on the amount of fat you can eat. Unsurprisingly, it's during this initial phase that most weight loss is achieved, although much of this is thought to be because of the loss of glycogen stores combined with water, and this is easily re-gained once carbs are re-introduced.

The plan encourages dieters to cut out processed, refined carbs as well as alcohol but allows the inclusion of red meat, butter, cream and cheese. The only fat Atkins suggests you avoid are the man-made trans fats typically found in spreads and processed foods. These trans fats have been linked to clogged arteries and an increased risk of heart disease and stroke.

Enjoying some fat in a healthy, balanced diet is important because it help promote our absorption of fat soluble vitamins like vitamin A, D, E and K, and certain fats are essential to health. These essential omega fats are needed in the diet for the manufacture of hormones and for a healthy nervous system.

More recent evidence is also suggesting that the saturated fat in dairy foods may be less harmful than we once thought. However, although Atkins places no limit on saturates, public health advice remains that we should limit our consumption to 20g of saturates daily. Choosing lower fat animal products like poultry, fish and lean cuts of pork would help towards this. In order to achieve your 5-a-day, any follower of the Atkins diet needs to understand which fruit and vegetable are low carb, so it's important to understand what is a starchy veg (those restricted by the diet) and those which are non-starchy (those which can be included). Good choices of non-starchy veg would be courgette, cucumber and leafy greens like spinach. Low carb fruits would include avocado and olives. Eating a wide range of fruit and veg not only allows us to get plenty of vitamins and fibre but also means we benefit from protective plant compounds like flavonoids and carotenoids which help fight heart disease, certain cancers and may help delay the signs of aging. Most health professionals believe that cutting out major food groups may be detrimental to long term health and in particular a high protein diet, like Atkins, if followed consistently over a long term may have an adverse effect on areas such as bone health, as well as renal function for those with an existing kidney condition.

THE ATKINS DIET

The Atkins diet is similar to a ketogenic diet as both emphasise the consumption of fat and protein but severely restrict carbohydrates. The body will turn to glycogen stores (carbohydrates) for energy first if supplies are plentiful. Ketogenic diets essentially force the body to switch from burning carbohydrates for energy to burning fat. This often has the desirable effect of weight loss, though high levels of ketones in the body can be problematic and may lead to a state known as ketosis.

The Atkins diet aims to help a person lose weight by limiting carbohydrates and controlling insulin levels. Dieters can eat as much fat and protein as they want.

The Atkins diet is designed to reduce carbohydrate intake significantly. The Atkins Diet has four core principles:

- to lose weight
- to maintain weight loss
- to achieve good health

- to lay a permanent foundation for disease prevention

The main reason for weight gain is the consumption of refined carbohydrates, or carbs, especially sugar, high fructose corn syrup, and flour.

When a person follows the Atkins Diet, their body's metabolism switches from burning glucose, or sugar, as fuel to burning stored body fat. This switch is called ketosis.

When glucose levels are low, insulin levels are also low, and ketosis occurs. In other words, when glucose levels are low, the body switches to using its fat stores, as well as dietary fat, for energy. In theory, this can help a person lose body fat and weight.

Before a person eats, their glucose levels are low, so their insulin levels are also low. When that person eats, their glucose levels rise, and the body produces more insulin to help it use glucose.

The glycemic index (GI) is a scale that ranks carbohydrates, or carbs, from 0 to 100, depending on how quickly they increase blood sugar levels after consumption, and by how much.

Refined carbs, such as white bread and candy, contain high levels of glucose. These foods have high GI scores, as their carbs enter the blood rapidly, causing a glucose spike.

Other types of carbs, such as beans, do not affect blood glucose levels so quickly or severely. They have a low glycemic load and score lower on the glycemic index.

Net carbs are the total carbs minus fiber and sugar alcohols. Sugar alcohols have a minimal effect on blood sugar levels. According to Dr. Atkins, the best carbs are those with a low glycemic load.

Fruits and grains are high in carbs, and a person on the Atkins diet restricts these, especially in the early stages. However, these foods are also good sources of vitamins, minerals, fiber, and antioxidants.

To make up for the lack of nutrient-rich foods, the Atkins diet encourages people to use vitamin and mineral supplements.

The Atkins diet may help a person lose weight. For many, losing weight will also reduce the risk of type 2 diabetes, cardiovascular disease, and other aspects of metabolic syndrome.

While a low carb approach may not work or be sustainable for everyone, clinical trials show that the Atkins diet results in similar or greater weight loss in those following it for at least 12 months compared to other options, such as the Mediterranean or DASH diets.

People who use medication for diabetes, cardiovascular disease, and other conditions should not stop taking these when they follow this or any other diet.

USING THE FAT IN THE BODY

If there is minimal carbs intake via the diet, ketosis will occur. During ketosis, the body will breakdown fat stores in the cells, resulting in the creation of ketones. These ketones then become available for the body to use as energy.

The Atkins diet is a low carb diet where the body burns more calories than on other diets because ketosis occurs. It is a kind of ketogenic diet, though protein intake is typically higher, and fat is lower in comparison to a traditional ketogenic diet.

HOW ATKINS DIET WORKS

THE ATKINS DIET: GETTING STARTED, STAYING FOCUSED

The Atkins Diet is an organized program for achieving permanent weight control through the intelligent consumption of carbohydrates. And there's more than weight loss at stake here: what really matters is your overall health and well being. In fact, many people who don't need to lose weight choose to follow the Atkins because of all the health benefits it provides.

Atkins is a four-phase lifetime eating plan that helps you:

- Achieve a carbohydrate awareness regarding quality and quantity of carbohydrates consumed
- Learn your individual threshold for carbohydrate consumption
- Incorporate vitamin and mineral supplementation and regular exercise

Here's what else you need to know about Atkins:

- Though certain guidelines must be followed, the Atkins is flexible, with a wide variety of choices to suit a variety of eating preferences and lifestyles.
- Atkins is not a one-size-fits-all approach—it is a customized eating plan that you will match to your unique metabolism. By learning your individual threshold for carbohydrate consumption, you can reach your ideal goal weight and stay there—without hunger pangs or feelings of deprivation.

THE FOUR PRINCIPLES OF ATKINS DIET

Atkins is based on four core principles, all backed by solid scientific research:

• **Weight loss**

• **Weight maintenance**

• **Good health and well-being**

• **Disease prevention**

THE FOUR PRINCIPLES

Let's take a closer look at the four principles of Atkins:

• **Weight Loss:**Both men and women who follow Atkins readily lose pounds and inches. If you're one of the very few who has a truly hard-core metabolic resistance to weight loss, there are ways to overcome the barriers that prevent a successful outcome.

• **Weight Maintenance:**Most low-fat, low-calorie diets may fail for one reason: hunger. Although many people can tolerate hunger for a while, very few can tolerate it for a lifetime. When you do Atkins, you feel satisfied by the foods you eat; you gradually find your effective individual level of carbohydrate intake, which is the tool that allows you to maintain a healthy weight for a lifetime.

• **Good Health and Well-Being:**With Atkins, you'll meet your nutritional needs by eating healthy, wholesome foods and omitting junk food. You'll find that this results in less fatigue—not just because you're losing pounds, but also because you will stabilize your blood sugar. When you do Atkins, you start feeling good long before they reach your goal weight.

• **Disease Prevention:** By following an individualized controlled-carbohydrate nutritional approach that results in lower insulin production, people at high risk for chronic illnesses such as cardiovascular disease, hypertension and diabetes will see a marked improvement in their health.

BENEFITS OF THE ATKINS DIET

The Atkins diet is becoming very popular nowadays and it has developed very many competitors who provide diets with similar principles. It is basically a diet that emphasizes on low carbohydrate intake and there are numerous diets from different firms which claim to be effective. These are a couple of the benefits of Atkins diet.

1. EFFECTIVE FOR WEIGHT LOSS

The intake of foods with low carbohydrates is very beneficial in any weight loss program. The Atkins diet usually helps an individual to lose weight without restricting their calorie intake. The end result is a much healthier and fit person.

2. IMPROVES BODY HEALTH

It has been proven that the consumption of the low carbohydrate Atkins diet increases good cholesterol in the body. This is especially important for people with diabetes since it helps in reducing the levels of glucose in the blood.

3. INCORPORATES DIFFERENT TYPES OF FOODS

This is one of the best benefits of Atkins diet that dieters are going to enjoy and thus motivate them to continue dieting. The Atkins diet is inclusive of some very tasty meals that the users can enjoy such as steak. Many people enjoy using the Atkins diet since it provides them freedom in comparison to other restrictive diets.

4. VERY SIMPLE TO USE

Once you have learnt the various carbohydrate counts present in different meals, you can start using the Atkins diet. It is highly advisable that you locate your own position on the provided carbohydrate chart because not every individual has the same qualities. Certain people have increased tolerance for the carbohydrates than others. When using the Atkins diet, you are going to find out your own carbohydrate level as well as how you can use that knowledge to your benefit.

However, people who use the Atkins diet over a long period of time usually suffer from fatigue and frequent migraines. The other disadvantage is rapid weight gain if you stop using this particular diet.

5. MAY NORMALIZE TRIGLYCERIDE AND CHOLESTEROL LEVELS

The Atkins diet is high in fat, specifically saturated fats that many fear contribute to heart problems. However, when saturated fat comes from healthy sources, such as grass-fed beef or coconut oil, it can actually be beneficial for raising HDL cholesterol levels and lowering risk factors for cardiovascular problems. Eating a balanced, unprocessed diet that results in healthy weight loss can also be vital in lowering LDL cholesterol and high triglycerides, which are tied to heart disease and heart attacks.

6. HELPS TREAT POLYCYSTIC OVARIAN SYNDROME (PCOS)

One of the leading risk factors for polycystic ovarian syndrome (PCOS) is having diabetes or being prediabetic, due to the effects of insulin on hormonal balance. PCOS is now the most common endocrine disorder affecting women of reproductive age. It is associated with problems like obesity, hyperinsulinemia, infertility and insulin resistance. While more research is still needed to draw conclusions, some studies have found that a low-carb ketogenic diet leads to significant improvement in PCOS symptoms— including weight, percent of free testosterone, LH/FSH hormone ratio and fasting insulin when followed for a 24-week period.

7. MAY REDUCE DEMENTIA RISK

Low-carb diets have been found to be beneficial for fighting cognitive problems, including dementia, Alzheimer's and narcolepsy. Researchers believe that people with the highest insulin resistance might demonstrate higher levels of inflammation and lower cerebral blood flow (circulation to the brain), therefore less brain plasticity.

THE 4 PHASES OF ATKINS DIET

The Atkins diet has four phases:

Phase 1: Induction

This first phase of the Atkins focuses on dramatic reduction of carbohydrate intake. It's the most restrictive phase of the program; it also results in the fastest weight loss, since your body will begin burning primarily fat for energy when sufficient calories from carbohydrates are not available. This occurs through a process called ketosis, which we'll talk about in more depth later in the course.

Doing Induction successfully requires that you stay on it for at least two weeks, although you can safely do it for months if you have a lot of weight to lose.

If you do not need to lose weight and you want to use this Phase to break addictions to junk food and sugar, you will need to make sure your calorie intake is very high to avoid weight loss. (Women should consume a minimum of 2,000 calories daily; men, 2,800 to 3,000 calories daily)

When you go into Induction you will:

• Limit carbohydrate consumption to 20 grams of Net Carbs (defined below) per day coming primarily from carbohydrates for a minimum of two weeks.

• Satisfy your appetite with foods that combine protein and fat, such as fish, poultry, eggs, lamb, pork and beef; eat limited amounts of hard cheeses (cheeses do contain some carbohydrates) .

• Consume a balance of healthy natural fats such as monounsaturated, polyunsaturated and saturated fats, but avoid manufactured trans fats (e.g. hydrogenated or partially hydrogenated oils).

• Consume carbohydrates in the form of nutrient-dense foods such as leafy green vegetables.

• Drink at least eight glasses of water daily.

Where Have All the Calories Gone?

Here's the first of a many pieces of good news you're going to get as you learn more about the Atkins Diet: You don't need to count calories at this point. You will naturally take in fewer calories because your appetite will be under control with sufficient amounts of protein and fat.

When you give your body too many carbohydrates to metabolize, it burns them for energy. But if you carefully control your carb intake, your body burns fat instead. And thatis the secret—if there is one—of the Atkins Diet.

As you read further, you'll see why that's true and how to determine what your net carb intake should be.

What' s a Net Carb?

The Atkins Diet works by restricting carbohydrates, which come from grains, legumes and other plant sources. But most carbohydrates contain fiber, which is not completely digested by the body. Fiber has a great effect on blood sugar, so these substances don't count as carbs on Atkins. So Net Carbs represent the total grams of carbohydrates minus grams of fiber. Net Carbs are the only carbs that you count when you do Atkins.

Successful completion of Induction means transitioning to the next phase: Ongoing Weight Loss.

As good as Induction is for quick, dramatic weight loss, it's important for you to understand that it's only the first Phase. Staying in Phase 1 for too long can become boring. Also, it can lead to a crash-diet mentality where you might assume it's okay to go back to eating anything, because you can always go back and lose the weight all over again by repeating Induction.

You can start with Phase 2 if you don't have a lot of weight to lose, don't want to lose weight at a slower pace, or you find Phase 1 too restrictive.

A person consumes less than 20 grams (g) of carbs each day. At this stage, carbs come mainly from salad and vegetables, which are low in starch.

Phase 2: Ongoing weight loss

When you switch to Ongoing Weight Loss (OWL), your rate of weight loss will naturally slow down. The first week on OWL, you will increase your daily carb intake from 20 to 25 grams; the following week you move to 30 grams of Net Carbs per day, and so on. You should increase intake on a weekly basis until your weight loss slows to one to two pounds each week.

During OWL you'll find out how many grams of carbs you can eat and still lose weight. This is called your personal carb balance.

When you go into OWL you can start adding back nutrient-dense foods like more non-starchy veggies (e.g., asparagus, broccoli); berries like raspberries and strawberries; nuts and seeds like hazelnuts and almonds; and soft cheeses (e.g., cottage cheese).

Phase 2 lasts until you're within 5 to 10 pounds of your weight goal. Successful completion of OWL includes transitioning to the third Phase of the program: Pre-Maintenance.

People gradually introduce nutrient-dense and fiber-rich foods as additional sources of carbs. These foods include nuts, seeds, low carb vegetables, and small amounts of berries. People can also add soft cheeses in this phase.

In phase 2, a person adds:

• 20–25 g of carbs per day during the first week

• 30 g of carbs during the second week

• 30 g each week until weight loss slows to 1–2 pounds a week

The aim of phase 2 is to find out how many carbs an individual can eat while continuing to lose weight. This phase continues until the individual is within 5–10 pounds of their target weight.

Phase 3: Premaintenance

When you're within 5 or 10 pounds of your target weight, it's time to move to Pre-Maintenance.

Now that your weight goal is in sight, the best strategy is to lose the last few pounds very slowly to start a permanently changed way of eating. This Phase lasts until you hit your target weight and maintain it for a month.

Each week in Pre-Maintenance you can add 10 more grams of Net Carbs to your daily allotment. As long as weight loss continues, you can gradually introduce foods such as lentils and other legumes, fruits other than berries, starchy vegetables and whole grains.

When you hit your goal weight and maintain it for at least a month, you've found your carb tolerance level. This is the level of carbohydrate intake at which you will neither gain nor lose weight, and is the key to the final phase, Lifetime Maintenance.

Dieters increase their carbs intake by 10 g each week. Weight loss will now be slow. They can start introducing legumes, such as lentils and beans, fruit, starchy vegetables, and whole grains to the diet.

People continue in this phase until they reach their target weight and maintain it for a month.

Phase 4: Lifetime maintenance

Once you've maintained your goal weight for a month, you've reached Lifetime Maintenance. Lifetime Maintenance is key to the Atkins Diet. In this Phase, the average number of daily grams of Net Carbs ranges from 40 to 120 per day, depending on your metabolism, age, gender, activity level and other factors. If you exercise regularly, you'll probably have a higher carb tolerance level.

In this stage, you will look great and feel great about your progress. But it's important for you to understand that losing weight is only a piece of the puzzle. Atkins isn't just about losing weight; it's also about maintaining health for life. Lifetime

Maintenance is designed to help you to stay healthy throughout your life.

The dieter starts adding a wider range of carbs sources, while carefully monitoring their weight to ensure it does not go up.

Net carb intake will vary between individuals, but it will usually be between 40–120 g a day.

However, these phases are a bit complicated and may not be necessary. You should be able to lose weight and keep it off as long as you stick to the meal plan below.

Some people choose to skip the induction phase altogether and include plenty of vegetables and fruit from the start. This approach can be very effective as well.

Others prefer to just stay in the induction phase indefinitely. This is also known as a very low-carb ketogenic diet (keto).

FOODS TO EAT AND TO BE AVOIDED

On Atkins you can continue to enjoy tasty foods with proteins, fats and fibre, so you'll feel satisfied and full. By eating foods that don't spike your insulin levels, your blood sugar is stabilised so you'll also experience more energy, your cravings disappear and you will feel less bloated.

From day one your eating plan will include green leafy vegetables alongside moderate protein sources such as chicken breast, steak or salmon. These are combined with healthy fats such as avocado, oils, butter, olives and cheese.

For vegetarians, Atkins is still a great way to follow a lower carb, balanced diet. Instead of getting your protein from meat, you can get it from kidney beans, black beans and chickpeas. Plus, you can try incorporating tofu, tempeh, eggs and cheese into your dishes. Fat sources include avocado, oils, butter and olives.

FOODS TO AVOID

You should avoid these foods on the Atkins diet:

- Sugar: Soft drinks, fruit juices, cakes, candy, ice cream, etc.
- Grains: Wheat, spelt, rye, barley, rice.
- Vegetable oils: Soybean oil, corn oil, cottonseed oil, canola oil and a few others.
- Trans fats: Usually found in processed foods with the word "hydrogenated" on the ingredients list.
- "Diet" and "low-fat" foods: These are usually very high in sugar.
- High-carb vegetables: Carrots, turnips, etc (induction only).
- High-carb fruits: Bananas, apples, oranges, pears, grapes (induction only).
- Starches: Potatoes, sweet potatoes (induction only).
- Legumes: Lentils, beans, chickpeas, etc. (induction only).

FOODS TO EAT

You should base your diet around these healthy foods.

- Meats: Beef, pork, lamb, chicken, bacon and others.

- Fatty fish and seafood: Salmon, trout, sardines, etc.

- Eggs: The healthiest eggs are omega-3 enriched or pastured.

- Low-carb vegetables: Kale, spinach, broccoli, asparagus and others.

- Full-fat dairy: Butter, cheese, cream, full-fat yogurt.

- Nuts and seeds: Almonds, macadamia nuts, walnuts, sunflower seeds, etc.

- Healthy fats: Extra virgin olive oil, coconut oil, avocados and avocado oil.

As long as you base your meals around a fatty protein source with vegetables or nuts and some healthy fats, you will lose weight. It's that simple.

BEVERAGES

Here there are some drinks that are acceptable on the Atkins diet.

• Water: As always, water should be your go-to beverage.

• Coffee: Many studies show that coffee is high in antioxidants and quite healthy.

• Green tea: A very healthy beverage.

Alcohol is also fine in small amounts. Stick to dry wines with no added sugars and avoid high-carb drinks like beer.

CAN BE EATEN

There are many delicious foods you can eat on the Atkins diet.

This includes foods like bacon, heavy cream, cheese and dark chocolate.

Many of these are generally considered fattening because of the high fat and calorie content.

However, when you're on a low-carb diet, your body increases its use of fat as an energy source and suppresses your appetite, reducing the risk of overeating and weight gain.

Most people feel that their appetite goes down on the Atkins diet.

They tend to feel more than satisfied with 3 meals per day (sometimes only 2).

However, if you feel hungry between meals, here are a few quick healthy snacks:

- Leftovers.

- A hard-boiled egg or two.

- A piece of cheese.

- A piece of meat.

- A handful of nuts.

- Some Greek yogurt.

- Berries and whipped cream.

- Baby carrots (careful during induction).

- Fruits (after induction).

ATKINS MENU FOR ONE WEEK

This is a sample menu for one week on the Atkins diet.

It's suitable for the induction phase, but you should add more higher-carb vegetables and some fruits as you move on to the other phases.

Monday

• Breakfast: Eggs and vegetables, fried in coconut oil.

• Lunch: Chicken salad with olive oil, and a handful of nuts.

• Dinner: Steak and veggies.

Tuesday

• Breakfast: Bacon and eggs.

• Lunch: Leftover chicken and veggies from the night before.

• Dinner: Bunless cheeseburger, with vegetables and butter.

Wednesday

• Breakfast: Omelet with veggies, fried in butter.

• Lunch: Shrimp salad with some olive oil.

• Dinner: Ground-beef stir fry, with veggies.

Thursday

• Breakfast: Eggs and veggies, fried in coconut oil.

• Lunch: Leftover stir fry from dinner the night before.

• Dinner: Salmon with butter and vegetables.

Friday

• Breakfast: Bacon and eggs.

• Lunch: Chicken salad with olive oil and a handful of nuts.

• Dinner: Meatballs with vegetables.

Saturday

• Breakfast: Omelet with various vegetables, fried in butter.

• Lunch: Leftover meatballs from the night before.

• Dinner: Pork chops with vegetables.

Sunday

• Breakfast: Bacon and eggs.

• Lunch: Leftover pork chops from the night before.

• Dinner: Grilled chicken wings, with some salsa and veggies.

Make sure to include a variety of different vegetables in your diet.

A simple Shopping List for the Atkins Diet.It's a good rule to shop at the perimeter of the store. This is usually where the whole foods are found.

Eating organic is not necessary, but always go for the least processed option that fits your budget.

- Meats: Beef, chicken, lamb, pork, bacon.

- Fatty fish: Salmon, trout, etc.

- Shrimp and shellfish.

- Eggs.

- Dairy: Greek yogurt, heavy cream, butter, cheese.

- Vegetables: Spinach, kale, lettuce, tomatoes, broccoli, cauliflower, asparagus, onions, etc.

- Berries: Blueberries, strawberries, etc.

- Nuts: Almonds, macadamia nuts, walnuts, hazelnuts, etc.

- Seeds: Sunflower seeds, pumpkin seeds, etc.

- Fruits: Apples, pears, oranges.

- Coconut oil.

- Olives.

- Extra virgin olive oil.

• Dark chocolate.

• Avocados.

• Condiments: Sea salt, pepper, turmeric, cinnamon, garlic, parsley, etc.

It's highly recommended to clear your pantry of all unhealthy foods and ingredients. This includes ice cream, sodas, breakfast cereals, breads, juices and baking ingredients like sugar and wheat flour.

THE 11 DIET SWAPS THAT MAKE THE LOW-CARB DIET EASY

Replace pasta with spiralised vegetables

Try making your own alternative to pasta at home by spiralizing courgette, carrot or other veg. You can buy a gadget to help you make perfect swirls or just use a grater. Serve with chicken or fish and make your own spicy tomato sauce or a tasty creamy sauce.

Get a chocolate hit that's low-carb

Swap your afternoon chocolate bar for an Atkins bar, which contains a fraction of the carbs yet tastes just as great (or even better!). A filling 60g Atkins bar contains 1-3g carbs, compared to 30-40g in a typical chocolate bar.

Control your coffee choice

Avoid high sugar milk from your local coffee shop and make your own version using unsweetened soya milk, espresso and a dollop of sugar-free whipped cream on top. A tall latte is typically around 17 grams sugar, compared to two grams for your home-made version!

Stick to wine

Alcohol can be loaded with carbs so avoid beer, cider and sugary cocktails and stick to wine. It's your choice whether you prefer red or white, but pinot noir is typically lower in carbs than other reds. For white, stick to crisp, dry wines for fewer carbs. Remember to drink water between each drink; not only it will stop you from getting a hangover but you'll feel fuller and less likely to give into cravings.

Do your own barbecue meat

Having a BBQ? Don't buy store-bought meats, which come with cereal fillers, or sugary marinades. Save pounds and lbs, by making your own BBQ feast. Skewer chicken pieces with vegetables, for healthy, colourful kebabs, or make your own burgers using mince meat, spices and a bit of chopped chilli and avoid the heavy burgers you find in shops.

Go no carb Mexican

Most Mexican food is great on Atkins with plenty of protein, guacamole, salsas and salads but use large lettuce leaves to wrap up the tasty fillings rather than carb-heavy tortillas.

Have a fry up without the carbs

By all, means enjoy a full English breakfast, but omit the carb heavy beans, hash browns and toast – and double up on bacon, eggs and mushrooms (the best bits!)

Cauliflower pizza is actually really nice

Might sound a little odd, but you'd never know you were eating cauliflower, and it's so easy to make. Just cut some cauliflower into florets, blend into small pieces, then mix with mozzarella, parmesan, seasoning, garlic and 2 eggs. Spread into a pizza shape on a baking sheet covered with baking powder, bake for 20 mins, then add the desired toppings and bake for a further 10 minutes.

Make the salad the main event

Salads can be great but can also be boring…don't just stick to limp lettuce, make yours a tasty treat by adding olives, feta, sliced avocado, sliced jalapenos, chorizo slices, crushed nuts and other low carb additions.

Don't get too hungry

Many people skimp on calories when trying to lose weight and it just doesn't work. On Atkins, we recommend three meals with two between-meal snacks. So your blood sugar levels stabilise and you never feel hungry. Try one of our tasty bars for one of your snacks for a mid-morning or afternoon treat.

Try an Atkins Bar

Atkins bars are a great way to snack between meals and not ruin your eating plan. They're low in sugar as well as carbs so are ideal for if you're out about on the go or need a pick me up pre- or post workout.

How to Follow the Atkins Diet when eating out

It's actually very easy to follow the Atkins diet at most restaurants.

1. Get extra vegetables instead of bread, potatoes or rice.

2. Order a meal based on fatty meat or fatty fish.

3. Get some extra sauce, butter or olive oil with your meal.

HOW THE ATKINS DIET IS BETTER THAN OTHER POPULAR DIETS

Atkins diet marginally better than rivals, Atkins and keto are two of the best-known low-carb diets.

Both stipulate a drastic reduction in high-carb foods, including sweets, sugary drinks, breads, grains, fruits, legumes, and potatoes.

Though these diets are similar, they have differences as well. The Atkins diet is one of the best-known diets worldwide. It's a low-carb, moderate-protein, high-fat diet.

Though Atkins has evolved to offer a variety of plans, the original version (now called Atkins 20) is still the most popular.

The keto diet

The keto, or ketogenic, diet is a very-low-carb, moderate-protein, high-fat diet plan.

It was first used to treat children who experienced seizures, but researchers discovered that it may benefit other people as well.

The goal of the keto diet is to get your body into the metabolic state of ketosis, during which it uses fat rather than sugar from carbs as its main energy source.

In ketosis, your body runs on ketones, which are compounds that are formed upon the breakdown of the fat in your food or the fat stored in your body.

To achieve and maintain ketosis, most people need to limit their total carb intake to 20–50 grams per day. Macronutrient ranges for the keto diet are typically under 5% of calories from carbs, 10-30% from protein, and 65-90% from fat.

Similarities and differences

Keto and Atkins share certain similarities but also differ greatly in some respects.

- Similarities

As they're both low-carb diets, Atkins and keto are alike in some ways.

In fact, Phase 1 (Induction) of the Atkins diet is similar to the keto diet, as it restricts net carbs to 25 grams per day. In doing so, your body likely enters ketosis and starts burning fat as its main source of fuel.

What's more, both diets may result in weight loss by decreasing the number of calories you eat. Many carbs — particularly refined carbs like sweets, chips, and sugary drinks — are high in calories and may contribute to weight gain.

Both Atkins and keto require you to eliminate these high-calorie, carb-rich foods, which makes it easier to cut calories and lose weight.

- Differences

Atkins and keto have certain differences as well.

While keto is a moderate-protein approach, with about 20% of calories coming from protein, the Atkins diet allows for up to 30% of calories from protein, depending on the phase.

Additionally, on the keto diet, you want to keep your body in ketosis by extremely limiting your carb intake.

On the other hand, the Atkins diet has you gradually increase your carb intake, which will eventually kick your body out of ketosis.

Due to this flexible carb limit, Atkins allows for a wider variety of foods, such as more fruits and vegetables and even some grains.

Overall, Atkins is a less restrictive approach, as you don't have to monitor ketones or stick to certain macronutrient targets to stay in ketosis.

Potential benefits

Though once considered unhealthy, low-carb diets have now been shown to offer various health benefits.

- Weight loss

Low-carb diets may result in more weight loss than other diet plans.

In a review of six popular diets, including Atkins, the Zone diet, the Ornish diet, and Jenny Craig, Atkins resulted in the most weight loss after six months .

A similar study found that Atkins was the most likely among 7 popular diets to result in meaningful weight loss 6–12 months after starting the plan.

Though more restrictive than Atkins, the keto diet may aid weight loss as well. Research indicates that being in ketosis decreases appetite, thereby removing one of the biggest barriers to weight loss — constant hunger.

Ketogenic diets also preserve your muscle mass, meaning that most of the lost weight is more likely to be a result of fat loss.

In one 12-month study, participants on a low-calorie keto diet lost about 44 pounds (20 kg) with few losses in muscle mass, compared to the standard low-calorie group, which only lost 15 pounds (7 kg).

Additionally, ketogenic diets maintain your resting metabolic rate (RMR), or the number of calories you burn at rest, whereas other low-calorie diets may cause your RMR to decrease.

- Blood sugar control

Research indicates that low-carb diets can benefit blood sugar control.

In fact, the American Diabetes Association recently revised the Standards of Medical Care, a document outlining how healthcare providers should manage and treat diabetes, to include low-carb diets as a safe and effective option for people with type 2 diabetes.

Low-carb diets have been shown to decrease the need for diabetes medications and improve levels of hemoglobin A1c (HgbA1c), a marker of long-term blood sugar control.

One 24-week study in 14 obese adults with type 2 diabetes on the Atkins diet found that in addition to losing weight, participants lowered their HgbA1c levels and decreased their need for diabetes medications.

Another 12-month study in 34 overweight adults noted that participants on a keto diet had lower HgbA1c levels, experienced more weight loss, and were more likely to discontinue diabetes medications than those on a moderate-carb, low-fat diet.

Other benefits

Research suggests that low-carb, higher-fat diets may improve certain heart disease risk factors.

Low-carb diets may reduce triglyceride levels and increase HDL (good) cholesterol, thereby decreasing the ratio of triglycerides to HDL cholesterol.

A high triglyceride-to-HDL ratio is an indicator of poor heart health and has been linked to increased heart disease risk.

A review including over 1,300 people found that those on the Atkins diet had greater decreases in triglycerides and more significant increases in HDL cholesterol than individuals following a low-fat diet.

Low-carb diets have also been associated with other benefits, including improved mental health and digestion.

WHAT YOU SHOULD KNOW BEFORE YOU BEGIN ATKINS DIET

Things You Should Know Before Starting the Atkins Diet

1. Atkins was the staple diet of the early 2000s.

Though Atkins began in 1972 when Robert C. Atkins released his book, Dr. Atkins' Diet Revolution, it didn't become crazy popular until the early 2000s, when he released his second book.

2. Krispy Kreme and the pasta industry were not fans.

The doughnut giant blamed Atkins and other low-carb diets like it for a huge drop in sales.

3. The key is to eat low carb, not low cal.

Atkins works by reducing sugar and carbs (which later turn into sugar) so that the body doesn't burn these for fuel but burns fat instead. In that sense, you're counting your net carb intake—AKA, those bites of bread and pasta you just can't resist—rather than count calories.

4. There's two diet plans to suit your needs.

If you follow Atkins, there are 2 plans to choose from: Atkins 20 and Atkins 40. With Atkins 20, you start by eating only 20 net carbs per day and eventually add more carbs (and food options) as you move through its four phases. This plan is recommended for people who have 40 or more pounds to lose.

With Atkins 40 you can eat, you guessed it, 40 net carbs per day. With this plan you eat three meals and two snacks per day, and you have way more food options. This option is good for people who have less than 40 pounds to lose, are breast feeding, or just need a little more variety in their meals.

5. Atkins lets you eat lots and lots of cheese.

A diet that lets you eat cheese? Yup, it exists. Atkins advocates eating both dairy and healthy fats, so you can keep munching on that fancy brie, or have yourself a little pat of butter—no problem (as long as you account for the net carbs, of course).

6. You'll have to pack on the protein.

Atkins is big on protein with every meal. In fact, at three 4- to 6-ounce servings on Atkins 40, it's a large part of your daily food intake. The good news is you can get your protein from lots of foods, including eggs, poultry, seafood, buffalo (hmmm), and even bacon.

7. You'll also have to put your alcohol behind lock and key.

Unfortunately, alcohol is not a part of either Atkins 20 or 40. Though the occasional glass of wine is no biggie, alcohol consumption slows down weight loss, so if you're really looking to lose weight, you should avoid drinking a whole bottle. Approved alcohols include: wine, rye, scotch, vodka, and gin—but lose the juice, tonic water, and non-diet soda, they'll add unwanted carbs and ruin your hard work.

8. Vegetarians and vegans can get in on the action too.

Atkins is an EOD (Equal Opportunity Diet) so non-meat eaters can follow the food plan by getting their protein from eggs, cheese, and soy products. Vegans can eat seeds, nuts, soy products, soy and rice cheeses, and high-protein grains like quinoa.

9. The diet has been recently corrected to include a lot more plants.

Atkins recently released a hip new version of its diet plan called Eco-Atkins. The new diet focuses on getting 31 percent of calories from plant proteins, 43 percent from plant fats and 26 percent from plant carbs, so basically this is the diet for vegetarians. There's little guidance on the diet (it doesn't even have an online presence), making it kind of hard to follow.

10. They have frozen meals and recipes galore to keep you on track.

Let's be real: Frozen meals are definite not the most appetizing thing in the world, but they do cut out the math of having to calculate net carbs yourself (they're printed on the box), and they're fast. Atkins has a variety of frozen meals, including breakfast options, a range of American options, and even global choices. My recommendation? Try the beef merlot or meatloaf—they're bomb. However, save yourself the disappointment and steer clear of the chicken options.

11. You can also get fresh meals delivered.

Not into frozen, but also not into cooking? That's cool. If you've got the cash, you can get fresh Atkins meals delivered to you. You can subscribe and get a personalized meal plan, or order a la carte.

12. Counting carbs? There's an app for that.

Atkins wouldn't make it in the 21st century if it didn't have a carb-counting app. The app functions like most others of its kind, but in addition to having the nutrition info for basically every grocery item on the planet, it includes data for Atkins products and recipes. So basically, you just type in words and never actually have to do math to figure out your carb intake, making dieting a no-brainer.

13. It's gonna get worse before it gets better.

If you're dieting, it means you're most likely really changing your eating habits, and that's obviously not going to be easy. People on Atkins tend to have initial some effects, including headaches, dizziness, weakness, fatigue and constipation. Of course, these side effects might occur with any diet, so it really is up to you: Is the gain worth the pain?

14. It may or may not have other health benefits.

Atkins marketing never fails to mention that aside from helping to lose weight, the diet plan also reduces risk for heart disease and diabetes.

15. It initially advocated unlimited cheese and meat.

Part of the reason why some doctors were initially skeptical of Atkins is because at first, it advocated eating cheese, meats, and fats liberally. Since then, the diet has undergone some changes, namely advocating for more moderation in dining on meat and dairy. Some experts are still not entirely convinced about a high-fat and protein diet, but little extensive research has been done.

16. Some prolific stars are fans of the diet.

Many stars have been rumored to use Atkins to maintain their weight.

17. It's kind of expensive.

Atkins, by virtue of making you eat fresh, non-processed food, is a pricey diet to maintain.

TIPS ABOUT HOW TO DO ATKINS DIET SUCCESSFULLY

Tips for Success on the Atkins Diet

Following these 16 tips will help you stay on track and get started on Atkins:

1. Understand what you are eating and how Atkins works. Atkins is all about eating right. You'll learn which foods your body needs to lose or maintain weight, how to easily reduce the amount of added sugar and other empty carbs and in your diet, how to understand what that Nutritional Facts label really says and more.

2. Atkins, customized for you. Depending on how much weight you have to lose, Atkins has a plan that will work for you: Atkins 20, the original plan that has you consuming 20 Net Carbs a day or Atkins 40, where you consume 40 grams of Net Carbs a day and a full range of food options.

3. Count your carbs. Understand what Net Carbs are and how to calculate them, using the handy Carb Counter in combination with the Acceptable Foods lists for your plan.

4. Be sensible, not obsessive, about portions. There's no need to count calories on Atkins, but you should use common sense. You probably could guess that too many calories will slow down weight loss, but too few will slow down your metabolism—and, therefore, weight loss. You only need worry about calories if, despite following Atkins to the letter, you cannot lose weight. Depending upon your height, age and metabolism, you may need to play with the following calorie ranges to lose weight: Women, should stick with 1,500–1,800 calories a day and men should stick with 1,800–2,200 calories per day.

5. Eat regularly. That's right, no starving! Regardless of which phase you're in, eat three regular-sized meals plus two snacks every day. Or, if you prefer, have four or five small meals throughout the day.Eating every few hours maintains blood sugar and energy levels and keeps your appetite under control. Eat until you're satisfied but not stuffed. Atkins has a full range of products,

including frozen meals, shakes, bars and treats that make it convenient and easy to stay on track.

6. Include protein in every meal. Make sure you are having 4 to 6 ounces of protein at breakfast, lunch and dinner. Men can have up to 8 ounces. You can choose eggs, meat (lean or fatty is fine), poultry; even marbled cuts of beef are fine. When leaner cuts are used, be sure to ensure enough of olive oil or other healthy oils on salads and cooked veggies.

7. Savor foods with natural fats. Fat makes food taste good and is filling so you eat less. In fact, dietary fat is key to the Atkins program, and to overall good health. All fats except manufactured trans fats (hydrogenated or partially hydrogenated oils) are a healthy part of Atkins.

8. Steer clear of added sugar. Added sugar comes in many forms and is found in most soft drinks and countless other foods. All are high in carbs and calories and empty of other nutrients. Instead, sweeten beverages with non-caloric sweeteners (stevia, sucralose—marketed as Splenda™— saccharin or xylitol.) Count each packet as 1

gram of Net Carbs and don't exceed three a day.

9. Eat veggies. Be sure to consume at least 12 to 15 grams of carbohydrates in the form of Foundation Vegetables each day. From the start, you'll meet the USDA's recommended intake of at least five daily servings of vegetables. You'll also be getting plenty of fiber, which plays a key role in blood sugar management, and, of course, regularity. Fiber also helps you feel full, and helps with weight control.

10. Enjoy eating—at home, in a restaurant, wherever. Unlike other diets that instill a fear of eating or require the purchase of expensive, pre-packaged meals, Atkins is all about eating delicious whole foods. You'll learn how to choose the right foods whether you're dining in or out, whether you're at a fast-food place or an ethnic restaurant, on the road for business or on vacation. Soon you'll know how to make the right choices and stay on track.

11. Drink up. Water and other fluids like tea and coffee (in moderation) encourage your body to let go of water weight—plus water

is just plain healthy. Aim for eight 8-ounce glasses each day.

12. Take daily supplements. In combination with a whole-foods diet, supplements are a good protocol on any weight loss program. Take a daily multivitamin with minerals, including potassium, magnesium and calcium, but without iron—unless you are iron deficient. Also omega-3s in the form of fish oil or an alternative is a good therapeutic tool.

13. Get moving. There are countless benefits to physical activity and exercise as a natural partner to a healthy diet. Brisk walking, swimming and other fun activities are an integral component of Atkins. And the more muscle you build, the more calories you'll burn. You may want to wait a couple of weeks after starting Atkins to begin a new fitness regimen—or ramp up your existing one. And if you have a lot of weight to lose, you may want to start slowly with short walks or water aerobics.

14. Track your successes. We're talking about both pounds and health indicators. Weigh and measure yourself at the chest, waist and hips once a week. Also, keep a

journal of food and fluid intake, as well as challenges and victories. Numerous studies indicate journal keepers are more successful at weight management than others. Get some baseline tests before you start Atkins—and 3 to 6 months later for follow up lipid levels. Prepare to be amazed at how much healthier they've become.

15. Get support from friends and family. Let the important people in your life know how they're doing and feeling. An Atkins buddy can share the ups and downs of their journey. Also, be sure to join the Community Forum at Atkins.com.

16. Plan ahead. Stock your kitchen with the right food and snacks. Decide on your meals before you go grocery shopping so you don't fall back on your old (high-carb) food choices.

The Wrong Way to Do Atkins

1. Misconception: Atkins can be used as a short-term or crash diet.

Reality: If you do Induction for two weeks to drop 10 pounds and then go back to your old way of eating, you will be treating it as a crash diet. But that goes against everything I recommend, and will lead to problems in the long run.

2. Misconception: You can lose weight doing Atkins, then return to your old way of eating.

Reality: Do this, and as with your past attempts, you will neglect to change those eating habits that ensure you always regain lost weight.

3. Misconception: You can focus only on losing weight and minimize the maintenance aspects.

Reality: Any weight loss program that does not flow into weight maintenance is doomed to failure. The eating plan you will follow during Lifetime Maintenance is likely to be something between your menu during the Induction phase and the way you ate before you started Atkins.

4. Misconception: You can eat any food so long you do not exceed 20 grams of carbs a day.

Reality: If you eat junk foods or other nutrient deficient carbohydrate foods instead of vegetables and other nutrient-dense foods, you will miss most of the benefits I write about and you certainly will not be fostering long-term health.

5. Misconception: You can use Atkins for weight loss, but you don't have to bother with exercise and supplements if you don't have any health problems.

Reality: If you don't supplement with vitanutrients and exercise regularly, you may take off pounds, but you will miss out on important health benefits. And everyone needs exercise: It is not related only to weight loss.

6. Misconception: You can just continue to do Induction until you lose all of your weight.

Reality: You will lose weight more quickly if you continue doing Induction, but you won't learn how to keep that weight off permanently if you don't move through the four phases. More important, you will miss out on the benefits of the phytochemicals present in health-promoting carbohydrate foods.

7. Misconception: You can go back to eating your favorite foods after you lose weight. Reality: Your favorite foods may well be your problem foods. Unless you acknowledge and learn how to deal with your addictions, you are doomed to regain your weight and fall back into the dangerous cycle of high blood sugar and overproduction of insulin.

8. Misconception: You can do Induction during the week and binge on weekends and still lose or maintain weight.

Reality: When you do Atkins during the week and then cheat on the weekends, for several days after your binge, you are no longer burning fat. At most, you could be in the fat-burning state for only three days each week. In addition, you may have overstimulated your insulin response, increasing the metabolic risk factors underlying your weight problem. Remember that when you burn fat, dietary fat is also being burned. However, if you combine high carbs with high fat-the typical American diet-you can be increasing your cardiovascular risks.

9. Misconception: You can do Atkins while following a low-fat regimen.

Reality: To encourage your body to burn its own stores of fat, you need to reduce the amount of carbohydrates you eat, meaning you need to eat primarily foods rich in protein and fat. Remember that essential fatty acids play a role in normal metabolic function. Fat also plays a role in stabilizing blood sugar and increasing satiety. If fat intake is too low, you will not burn fat aggresively. Moreover, excess protein converts to glucose and can keep fat from becoming the primary fuel.

8 WEEKS ATKINS DIET MEAL PLAN FOOD YOU CAN ENJOY AND RECIPES FOR EACH PHASE

Anyone who is committed to doing Atkins properly needs to follow these rules to the letter. Remember that it takes two to three days for the body to switch to fat burning. One cheat and you're back to a glucose-burning metabolism. You can lose the effects of two or three days of fat burning with one cheat. So if you have the misguided belief that you can do Atkins all week and then indulge over the weekend, don't expect to see dramatic results.

Now to the meal plans. Follow this menu for the first week, then repeat it for the second week.

Meal Plans for the Atkins Diet

The types of meals that you should be eating will vary depending upon which stage of the diet you are at: Induction, Ongoing Weight-loss, Pre-maintenance or Maintenance.

Menu for the Induction Stage

Breakfast:

• Ham or bacon with eggs (fried or scrambled) and, to drink, decaffeinated tea or coffee.

Lunch:

• Bacon cheeseburger (making sure you serve it without the bun to avoid the carbohydrates) accompanied by a small salad and a glass of water.

Dinner:

• Prawn cocktail as a starter – the sauce should be made from mustard and mayonnaise.

• Clear consommé – this is a specialised kind of light soup made mainly from a kind of refined stock. This can be quite tricky to make so, unless you are particularly handy in the kitchen, you may prefer to search your local supermarket for a good, low carbohydrate brand Meat (choose any from the following: a steak, chops, a portion of fish, fowl or a roast) to be served with a salad.

• Sugar free jelly accompanied by a small serving of whipped cream (make sure this is also sugar free) for dessert.

Menu for the Ongoing Weight-loss Stage

Breakfast:

• Cheese omelette to be accompanied by some bran based crisp bread (to an amount containing carbohydrate to the value of 2 grams).

• To drink - decaffeinated tea or coffee and also 3 ounces of tomato juice

Lunch:

• A chicken, cheese, ham and egg salad. For the dressing keep it simple with an oil and vinegar based dressing.

• Herbal iced tea.

Dinner:

• A seafood salad.

• Poached salmon with a small portion of vegetables (avoid root vegetables to minimise your carbohydrate intake).

• A small portion of strawberries for dessert with double cream (unsweetened).

Menu for the Pre-maintenance and Maintenance Stages

Breakfast:

• Cheese and spinach omelette

• Half of one cantaloupe

• Bran based crisp bread with butter (to an amount containing carbohydrate to the value of 4 grams)

• Decaffeinated tea or coffee to drink

Lunch:

- Roast chicken accompanied by a small portion of vegetables and a salad. Try a green salad with a creamy garlic dressing

- Soda water to drink

Dinner:

- French onion soup to start

- Salad with onions, tomatoes and carrots with a dressing (without carbohydrate in it)

- Veal chops (these can be breaded, but not too heavily as this will contain carbohydrates) accompanied by a small portion of vegetables and half of a jacket potato topped with sour cream and chives

- A small portion of fresh fruit dessert compote

- 1 glass of dry wine (or, if you prefer, two white wine spritzers – this is the old fashioned kind with soda water rather than the modern version of the spritzer served with lemonade)

More Simple Meal Ideas with Atkins

There are plenty of meals which can complement your Atkins diet. Below are some ideas to get you started.

• Bacon, celery, walnut and avocado salad

• Thai coconut curry

• Chilli and pepper marinated steak

• Chicken kebabs with peanut dipping sauce

• Beef and mushroom skewers

• Pork in a creamy paprika sauce

• Stuffed, baked chicken wrapped in parma ham

• Baked marrow stuffed with cheeses

• Haddock stuffed with leek and spinach sauce

• Tandoori chicken skewers

• Lemon seafood salad

• Large mushrooms stuffed with goats cheese

• Eggs Benedict accompanied by hollandaise sauce

- Pork with a stilton based sauce to accompany

- Vegetable curry

ONE-WEEK INDUCTION MENU

Monday

BREAKFAST

- Two scrambled eggs
- Two turkey sausages

LUNCH

- Greek salad made with Romaine lettuce, half a tomato, feta cheese, olives and dill vinaigrette Small can of tuna

DINNER

- Veal Scallops with White Wine Caper Sauce*

- Sauteed spinach Gelatin dessert made with sucralose topped with whipped cream

SNACK

- Controlled carb strawberry shake

Tuesday

BREAKFAST
- Crustless Quiche*
- Two tomato slices

LUNCH
- Chicken salad served over chopped cucumber, radishes and watercress

DINNER
- Maple Mustard-Glazed Salmon*
- Sauteed broccoli with red pepper
- Small green salad with vinaigrette

SNACK
- Ten to twenty olives

Wednesday

BREAKFAST
- Smoked salmon and cream cheese roll-ups Two hard-boiled eggs

LUNCH
- Homemade Chicken Soup*

DINNER
- Broiled steak Oven-Fried Turnips*
- Arugula and Boston lettuce salad

SNACK
- Turkey, Romaine lettuce, mayonnaise roll-up

Thursday

BREAKFAST
- Western omelette with green salsa

LUNCH
- Vegetable broth with shredded white radish Shrimp salad over greens

DINNER
- Turkey Cutlets with Green Peppercorn Sauce* Cauliflower-Leek Puree*
- Gelatin dessert made with sucralose topped with whipped cream

SNACK
- One ounce Swiss cheese

Friday

BREAKFAST
- Two ounces cream cheese sprinkled with cinnamon and flaxseeds
- Two Bran-a-Crisp crackers

LUNCH
- Chef's salad with blue cheese dressing

DINNER
- Pork burgers Creamy Red Cabbage Slaw*
- Broiled portobello mushrooms with sesame oil

SNACK
- Mocha granita

Saturday

BREAKFAST
- Whitefish salad
- Two tomato slices

LUNCH
- Ham, spinach and cheese omelette
- Mixed green salad

DINNER
- Herbed-Roast Chicken with Lemon*
- Buttered green beans
- Italian Almond Cream*

SNACK
- Celery stuffed with Roasted Garlic and Vegetable Dip*

Sunday

BREAKFAST
- One and a half slices Zucchini Nut Bread* Two ounces cream cheese

LUNCH
- Broiled cheeseburger
- Large mixed green salad with two tomato slices

DINNER
- Cajun Pork Chops*
- Sauteed kale with garlic

SNACK
- Controlled carb vanilla shake

HOW THE ATKINS SYSTEM OF EATING CAN BE ADAPTED TO YOUR INDIVIDUALS NEEDS, EVEN PROVIDING YOU WITH TASTY DIABETIC-FRIENDLY RECIPES

For many, cutting out and minimising carbohydrate intake can be very difficult. There are many ways that you can try and make this a little easier however.

• The Atkins' diet has many tips on how to avoid carbohydrates and also additional helpful substitutes.

• You can order substitute products from the Atkins diet, such as Atkins bake mix, which reduce the carbohydrate content of your meals.

• The above reduced-carbohydrate bake mix minimises the carbohydrate content of all your baking so you can have cakes, breads, etc.

• Use sugar substitutes instead of regular sugar which should have less 'food energy'. Be sure to check the packets though to make sure this is the case – some substitutes are better than others.

• Search your local stores for controlled-carbohydrate pasta so that you can still enjoy your favourite Italian dishes from time to time.

• Use reduced-carbohydrate bread instead of regular brands. By doing this you can still enjoy a sandwich or two while you are on your diet.

• Sometimes this high-protein diet can become quite monotonous if you do not know how to vary your meals. Experiment with different ways of cooking things – use different spices and seasonings to add variety and interest to potentially similar meals. However be careful that you take note of the ingredients that you use when making your sauces. Ingredients such as refined white flour, honey and sugar can impede your weight loss when following the Atkins diet.

If you are finding it difficult to lose weight, or would like to lose more, then the above areas might provide you with some indication as to either where you are going wrong or where there are areas that you can reduce your carbohydrate intake even more.

ATKINS DIET FOR VEGETARIANS

The Atkins diet is much harder for vegetarians because meat proteins are an integral part of the diet and the suggested meal plans. It is likely that vegetarians will have much less successful results than those who eat meat, and involve more planning and care, so you may wish to look into alternative diet plans. If you are positive that you wish to go on the Atkins diet you should consult with your doctor or nutritionist first. It is likely that your meal plans will feature eggs and cheese heavily in order for you to consume sufficient amounts of protein.

THE ATKINS DIET AND VEGANS

The advice for vegetarians as above is relevant here, however it is likely that vegans will have to look for an alternative diet as you obviously will not have the protein sources listed above as options.

Vegan diets contain too much carbohydrate and it is extremely unlikely that you would be able to make a success of your Atkins diet in combination with this.

IDEAS TO FACILITATE YOUR VEGETARIAN ATKINS DIET

The following tips should help you to get you started on your vegetarian version of the Atkins diet.

• Research the traditional Atkins diet in detail. Make a note of any potential areas you will need to be aware of, for example keeping your protein levels up by increasing the quantity of cheese, tofu and egg you consume to make up for the fact you are not eating meat.

• Ensure that you check the labels of what you eat to minimise the amount of carbohydrates you consume, particularly in the first weeks of your Atkins diet when carbohydrate consumption should be as low as possible. The carbohydrates you do eat should come from berries, seeds, fresh vegetables and small amounts of fruit and nuts. Processed foods, sugar and white flour should all be removed from your diet. Remember that, while you do need to keep your protein intake up, foods such as cheese and tofu do contain some carbohydrate so you should take this into consideration when calculating your carbohydrate consumption.

• The fact that your sources of protein already up your carbohydrate intake means that you will have to be even more careful than meat eaters of the vegetables and fruits, etc. that you eat to ensure you are consuming those with the lowest carbohydrates in. This will allow you to try and even out and make up for the carbohydrates contained in your protein sources.

• After you have restricted your carbohydrate intake as much as possible, during the later stages of the diet, you can then very slowly reintroduce foods which have a higher carbohydrate concentration such as oats, cous cous, barley and vegetables with over 10 per cent carbohydrates in, most root vegetables for example.

• If you are comfortable including fish in your diet then this is a useful way of complementing your Atkins diet. This will add variety to your meals and also reduce the intake of carbohydrates instead which will hinder you sticking to the diet properly and, in doing so, also hinder your weight loss.

The stricter your vegetarian diet is, the harder it will be to stick to the Atkins diet. Protein is a very large part of the Atkins diet and so avoiding meat, and even fish, limits your options greatly.

Anyone should consult a health professional, nutritionist or medical practitioner before embarking upon any new nutrition plan or a drastic change in diet. If however you are a vegetarian this is even more applicable advice to ensure that you get the best out of your new diet plan whilst still getting the necessary nutrients.

ATKINS DIET SIDE EFFECTS

Typical side effects usually experienced by following the Atkins Diet.

There are many side effects that people tend to experience while following the Atkins diet. Some are just a short term inconvenience; however, some experts believe that the Atkins diet can also have a more long term detrimental effect on your health.

Short Term and Instant Side Effects of Atkins

There are various side effects which people can experience while following the Atkins diet. Different people experience different variations and combinations of the below symptoms shortly after beginning the Atkins diet:

• Fatigue

• Dizziness and generally feeling weak

• Insomnia

• Nausea

• Halitosis

• Constipation

Causes of These Short Term Side Effects

Any sudden, drastic change in diet can cause your body to react and in doing so cause different side effects. These may be very different for different people, however it is likely that you will experience at least a couple of the above symptoms. The symptoms of fatigue and feeling weak are a result of your body altering the energy source it uses. With the decrease in carbohydrate intake (its preferred energy source) your body must find other energy sources to use which can often make you feel lethargic, weak and sluggish. As you and your body get used to this change you will not experience these symptoms as much.

LONG TERM SIDE EFFECTS OF ATKINS

Much research has been done into whether the Atkins diet has more serious long-term side effects. While much of this research is inconclusive, many believe that the Atkins diet can have quite a detrimental effect upon your health, particularly if followed over a long period of time. Many believe that the likelihood of having or experiencing the following is much increased by being on the Atkins diet for any length of time:

• Heart disease

- Cancer

- Osteoporosis

- Premature aging

- Cataracts

- Kidney problems

- Weak bones

CAUSES OF THESE LONG TERM SIDE EFFECTS

These side effects are generally agreed to be as a result of the Atkins diet's reliance on what is essentially quite an imbalanced diet. The fact that many key nutrients do not feature in the diet is a cause of concern for many experts. Dr. Atkins emphasises the importance of taking vitamins and other supplements to make up for this. However most nutritionists agree that taking pills to get these nutrients is no substitute for consuming the correct foods to get them naturally. The importance of dairy in your diet cannot be underestimated for the benefits it provides your body, specifically in ensuring your bones are strong and healthy.

How to Minimise these Side Effects

The best way to minimise these side effects is to do as much research as possible in advance. Similarly you should consult at length with your medical practitioner and a dietician or nutritionist. By learning all of the facts and risks then you can embark upon your diet as healthily as possible and taking as many precautions as possible.

ATKINS & ATHLETES

Athletes require a great deal of energy in order to perform to their optimum level. The best energy source for the body comes from carbohydrates. This is because this is the only energy source that is stored as glycogen in your muscles. Without this energy source and its conversion in your muscles, athletes are unlikely to perform as well as they might otherwise be able to and they will also probably experience high levels of fatigue.

Given the amount of exercise that you do as an athlete, it is likely that the best diet for you is to observe the traditional balanced diet with plenty of fruits and vegetables. This should also include plenty of carbohydrates to sustain your volume of physical exertion. By incorporating some protein and whole foods and avoiding processed and junk foods you should still feel satisfied after meals and maintain a healthy weight and lifestyle.

If you are an athlete and you still wish to reduce your body fat percentage then it is recommended that you consult a nutritionist who specialises in sports nutrition. In this way they should be able to advise you so you can lose weight without compromising your performance.

HOW TO EAT LOW-CARB ON A BUDGET

If you're undertaking a new way of eating, such as a low-carb diet, you're probably wondering how your grocery bill will be affected. However, changing how you eat doesn't have to be a major monetary investment.

Buying more or less of specific foods, beverages, and other low-carb pantrystaples don't necessarily break the bank. Here are a few tips and tricks for eating low-carb on a budget.

Budget Basics

Even if you're not following a specific diet, being aware of the cost of groceries and trying to stick to a budget is a common experience for many shoppers. If you're on a low-carb diet, you'll also want to factor in the nutritional value of the foods you buy as well as eating a varied, balanced, diet.

Convenience, prep, and cooking requirements are also likely to influence your decisions when you're shopping and planning meals.

• The great news is that Atkins encourages the consumption of dietary fat and fattier cuts of meat are often the cheapest! So cuts like pork belly, 20% fat minced beef and chicken legs or thighs are much cheaper than pork chops, lean beef or skinless chicken breasts.

• Vegetables are great on Atkins and they are very often on sale in supermarkets. If so, buy in bulk and freeze the veg you don't use. I often buy a huge cauliflower when it's on offer and steam it all and then freeze the half I don't use. Then you can use the rest whether it's to make a cauli-pizza base, cauliflower cheese or adding to soups or stews.

• This is great for foods that are seasonal too, such as celeriac. This is a must in my house as I enjoy celeriac chips & mash; instead of starchier potato. So I buy it in season and freeze for when it's not available in my local supermarket.

• Local markets are also a great way to eat on a budget as they are often much cheaper than supermarkets, especially for meat, fish and fresh produce. So visit your local market, even if it's once a month, and stock up on essentials.

• Shop around! As well as your local market, try getting some of your shopping from stores like Aldi or Lidl. I've found their fruit & vegetable section to be excellent and much cheaper than the larger supermarkets. They also have great deals on low carb staples like flaxseeds and avocados.

• Buy frozen, if the vegetables you like are cheaper in their frozen form then go ahead. Just check the label as, unbelievably, some veg may have added sugar!

• Buy in bulk and portion your food into individual servings. This works well for great savings on protein like buying a whole side of salmon and then split into 8 or so servings and freeze. Much, much cheaper than buying individual portions.

• Eggs are a super food and so cheap! So stock up on free range eggs and you'll be getting a great source of protein and other nutrients for a fraction of the price of other protein rich foods.

• If you cook up double the portion size of your dinner-time meal then you'll have leftovers for lunch the next day which can save you ££s. It's much better to have a portion of low carb curry for your lunch, rather than a boring old sandwich!

• Don't feed the family any differently. Atkins friendly meals can be so tasty but just skip the starchy side from your plate. For instance, if you have pork belly with roasted veg, give yourself cheesy cauliflower instead of mashed potato that you may serve to the rest of the family.

LOW CARB DINING OUT STRATEGIES

Everybody likes going out to eat, and there are plenty of easy ways to enjoy a night out while staying true to your low carb goals. Regardless if you're on an Atkins plan or a similar keto diet, there are plenty of great options that are low in carbs and big in flavor. Both Atkins and keto activate your body's fat-burning metabolism by restricting carbs, so people following either diet will be looking for the same types of meal choices. If you're planning a night out, here are some keto friendly restaurants and menu picks:

Olive Garden

Topping off our list of keto restaurant options is the Italian staple, Olive Garden. If you are in the mood for seafood, we recommend the Herb-Grilled Salmon (460 calories, 28g total fat, 8g carbs, 4g fiber, and 43g protein). This fish filet is bursting with flavor as it is grilled to perfection and topped with garlic herb butter. It also comes with a side of delicious parmesan garlic broccoli. If fish isn't your thing, we recommend giving the tasty Parmesan-Crusted Zucchini (90 calories, 7g total fat, 5g carbs, 1g fiber, and 4g protein).

Chili's

Chili's, the home of flavorful Tex-Mex and American cuisine, is a great spot for something that isn't easily replicated at home. This bar and grill provides several options for those of us eating keto at restaurants. If you're in the mood for some Mexican flavors and spices, we recommend ordering the Chicken or Steak Fajitas (440/640 calories, 14/38g fat, 21/21g carbs, 3/3g fiber, and 59/55g protein) and enjoying without the tortillas or toppings. Instead of getting rice on the side, a double order of vegetables will be a great complement. We suggest boxing half of it to-go for lunch the next day to cut down on carbs. If you're not in the mood for Mexican on your night out, you're in luck! The House BBQ Ribs are another keto friendly option. A half rack of ribs without sauce will account for 720 calories, 53g total fat, 11g carbs, 1g fiber, and 49g protein.

Buffalo Wild Wings

Wings, beer, sports, and low carb choices. That's why Buffalo Wild Wings is one of our favorite keto restaurant options. Now, we can't recommend you grab a beer, but the snack size Traditional Wings with Medium Sauce (390 calories, 23g fat, 0g fiber, 1g carbs, and 44g protein) should do the trick! These wings will taste great while keeping you on pace to meet your keto goals. We also advise you to check out the BWW nutritional guides, as many other sauces and dry rubs are low in carbs!

Carrabba's

Get your Italian night on with another keto eating out option, Carrabba's. Our first choice would be the Tuscan Grilled Filet (590 calories, 44g total fat, less than 1g carbs, 0g fiber, and 47g protein). This juicy piece of meat is loaded with flavor while low in carbs. Another great option is the Pollo Rosa Maria (620 calories, 37g total fat, 4g carbs, 1g fiber, and 65g protein). Grilled chicken is stuffed with creamy fontina cheese and cured prosciutto, then topped with mushrooms and basil lemon butter. Make sure to get vegetables as a substitution to pasta on the side!

The Cheesecake Factory

A place filled with desserts can't possibly have low carb or keto restaurant options, can it? Of course, it can! The Cheesecake factory is a fantastic keto friendly restaurant. With several options to choose from, we recommend the Pan Seared Branzino with Lemon Butter (1130 calories, 93g fat, 22g carbs, 5g fiber, and 50g protein). This rich Mediterranean sea bass will hit the spot!

Red Robin

Red Robin is the home of fresh, fire-grilled burgers. Not only their food is packed and full of flavor, but it is also perfect for a keto or low carb lifestyle. The Wedgie™ Burger

(560 calories, 35g total fat, 22g carbs, 5g fiber, and 40g protein) is our go-to. This lettuce wrapped burger is topped with smoked bacon, house-made guacamole, tomatoes, and red onions. Who needs fries when your burger comes with a side salad? This meal is perfect for anyone trying to fulfill their Atkins or keto goals.

Red Lobster

If you're in the mood for some seafood on your night out, Red Lobster is a delicious keto restaurant option for you. The steamed Live Maine Lobster (440 calories, 34g fat, 0g carbs, 0g fiber, and 33g protein) has zero carbs (nice!) and is full of protein. If you're feeling surf & turf and are able to still meet your daily goals with some added carbs, you can't go wrong with The Rock Lobster & 12 of NY Strip Steak Combo (1,250 calories, 83g fat, 27g carbs, 4g fiber, and 97g protein).

A Few Tips For Going Keto At Restaurants:

Now that you know which keto friendly restaurants exist, it's time to get out and treat yourself. If you're going out for dinner at a restaurant that's not on this list, we have a few tips to keep in mind when eating out keto:

1. Plan ahead! If you're going out to eat, check the menu online ahead of time. You can also ask for nutrition information when you arrive. By law, restaurants must have that information available, making it easier than ever to make smart choices.

2. Meat and veggie options are your friends! These will typically be your best bet for lowcarb and protein-rich food.

3. Condiments like ketchup, BBQ sauce, and honey mustard tend to be high in sneaky carbs. If you need to add flavor, we recommend yellow mustard, ranch dressing, hot sauce, or butter.

4. Many entrées are served with a starch on the side, so opt for a side salad instead.

5. Don't be afraid to ask the waiter or waitress about keto friendly or low carb options!

ATKINS LOW CARB RECIPES

LOW CARB BREAKFAST RECIPES

Almond and Coconut Muffin in a Minute Recipe

Prep Time: 3 Minutes
Style:American
Cook Time: 1 Minutes
Phase: Phase 2

* Any adjustments made to the serving values will only update the ingredients of that recipe and not change the directions.
9.9g Protein, 19.2g Fat, 2.9g Fiber, 231.6kcalCalories, 3.7g Net Carbs.

INGREDIENTS
• 2 tablespoons Almond Meal Flour
• 1 teaspoon Coconut flour, high fiber
• 1 teaspoon Sucralose Based Sweetener (Sugar Substitute)

- 1/2 teaspoon Cinnamon
- 1/4 teaspoon Baking Powder (Straight Phosphate, Double Acting)
- 1/8 teaspoon Salt
- 1 large Egg
- 1 teaspoon Extra Virgin Olive Oil
- 1 tablespoon Sour Cream

DIRECTIONS

1. Place all dry ingredients in a coffee mug. Stir to combine.

2. Add the egg, oil, and sour cream. Stir until thoroughly combined.

3. Microwave for 1 minute. Use a knife if necessary to help remove the muffin from the cup, slice, butter, eat. For best results, eat immediately.

Note: Almond Meal from whole almonds is preferred for this recipe. Your MIM can be toasted once it's cooked and topped with cream cheese if you like. Replace the cinnamon with other spices, sugar-free syrup or 1/2 tsp unsweetened cocoa (net carb count will be .2g higher). Change the shape by making it in a bowl.

COOKING TIP: Try adding a small amount of almond or coconut extract to boost their flavors!

Almond Muffin in a Minute Recipe

Prep Time: 3 Minutes
Style:American
Cook Time: 1 Minutes
Phase: Phase 2

* Any adjustments made to the serving values will only update the ingredients of that recipe and not change the directions.
12.3g Protein, 23.5g Fat, 3.6g Fibre, 276.9kcalCalories, 4.5g Net Carbs.

INGREDIENTS
• 1/4 cup Bob's Red Mill Almond Meal/Flour (1/4 cup is 28g)
• 1 teaspoon No Calorie Sweetener
• 1/4 teaspoon Baking Powder (Straight Phosphate, Double Acting)
• 1 dash Salt
• 1/2 teaspoon Cinnamon
• 1 large Egg (Whole)
• 1 teaspoon Canola Vegetable Oil

DIRECTIONS

1. Place all dry ingredients in a coffee mug. Stir to combine.

2. Add the egg and oil. Stir until thoroughly combined.

3. Microwave for 1 minute. Use a knife if necessary to help remove the muffin from the cup, slice, butter, eat.

Note: Your MIM can be toasted once it's cooked and topped with cream cheese if you like. Replace the cinnamon with other spices, sugar-free syrup or 1/2 tsp unsweetened cocoa (net carb count will be .2g higher). Add a tablespoon of sour cream for a moister MIM. Change the shape by making it in a bowl.

COOKING TIP :Stirring the dry ingredients is a very important step to make sure your MIM bakes evenly.

Keto Almond Protein Pancakes

Prep Time: 5 Minutes
Style:American
Cook Time: 10 Minutes
Phase: Phase 2
Difficulty: Moderate

* Any adjustments made to the serving values will only update the ingredients of that recipe and not change the directions.
21.9g Protein, 9.1g Fat, 1.3g Fiber, 187.4kcalCalories,Net Carbs 3.2g.

INGREDIENTS
• 2 ounces Vanilla Whey Protein
• 1/4 cup Almond Meal Flour
• 3 tablespoons Whole Grain Soy Flour
• 1 teaspoon Baking Powder (Straight Phosphate, Double Acting)
• 3 large Eggs (Whole)
• 1/3 cup Large or Small Curd Creamed Cottage Cheese

DIRECTIONS
Top these naturally keto and low carb almond flour pancakes with almond butter, sugar-free syrup, or toasted almonds, if desired.

1. Mix the protein powder (1oz is about 4 Tbsp), almond meal, soy flour and baking powder together. Whisk the eggs, then blend together with the cottage cheese (substitute cream cheese if cottage cheese is not on your accepted foods list).

2. Heat a large nonstick skillet or griddle over medium heat. Lightly grease with butter or canola oil.

3. Using about 1/4 cup per pancake, drop batter onto the skillet. When bubbles begin to form in the middle of each pancake, turn over and cook another 2 minutes or until firm.

4. Repeat, keeping pancakes warm in the oven.

COOKING TIP: Add blueberries to the batter to add a fruit serving to this low carb breakfast or post workout meal (just pay attention to net carbs whenever you add ingredients).

Almond Protein Pancakes with Blueberries Recipe

Prep Time: 5 Minutes
Style:American
Cook Time: 10 Minutes
Phase: Phase 2
Difficulty: Moderate

* Any adjustments made to the serving values will only update the ingredients of that recipe and not change the directions.
24g Protein, 13.9g Fat, 4.1g Fiber, 256.5kcalCalories, Net Carbs 6.3g.

INGREDIENTS
• 2 tablespoons Blanched Almond Flour
• 3/4 large Egg (Whole)
• 1 1/2 tablespoons Whole Grain Soy Flour
• 1/4 teaspoon Baking Powder (Straight Phosphate, Double Acting)
• 1/2 ounce Large or Small Curd Creamed Cottage Cheese
• 2 tablespoons Vanilla Whey Protein
• 1/4 cup Fresh Blueberries

DIRECTIONS
1. Combine the almond flour, protein powder, soy flour and baking powder

together. Stir in the beaten egg and cottage cheese until blended.

2. Heat a large nonstick skillet or griddle over medium heat. Lightly grease with butter or canola oil.

3. Using about 1/4 cup per pancake, drop batter onto the skillet. When bubbles begin to form in the middle of each pancake, turn over and cook another 2 minutes or until firm.

4. Serve with blueberries Or add blueberries to the pancake batter before cooking.

COOKING TIP :Whether you're feeding a family or cooking for one, you can update the serving settings above to reveal the required amount of ingredients.

Almond Raspberry Smoothie Recipe

Prep Time: 5 Minutes
Style:American
Cook Time: Minutes
Phase: Phase 2
Difficulty: Easy

* Any adjustments made to the serving values will only update the ingredients of that recipe and not change the directions.
18.2g Protein, 13.7g Fat, 6.9g Fiber, 259.4kcalCalories, 10.3g Net Carbs.

INGREDIENTS
• 4 ounces Greek Yogurt - Plain (Container)
• 1/2 cup Red Raspberries
• 20 each wholes Blanched & Slivered almonds
• 1/2 cup Pure Almond Milk - Unsweetened Original

DIRECTIONS
Feel free to come up with your own combination of other berries and nuts for this protein-packed smoothie. If you use frozen raspberries, make sure they contain no added sugar.
Combine the yogurt, raspberries, almonds and almond milk in a blender and purée until smooth and creamy.

COOKING TIP: Whether you're feeding a family or cooking for one, you can update the serving settings above to reveal the required amount of ingredients.

Almond-Pineapple Smoothie Recipe

Prep Time: 5 Minutes
Style:American
Cook Time: Minutes
Phase: Phase 3
Difficulty: Easy

* Any adjustments made to the serving values will only update the ingredients of that recipe and not change the directions.
10.7g Protein, 17.3g Fat 3.9g Fiber 275.7kcalCalories, 16.1g Net Carbs.

INGREDIENTS
• 1/2 cup (8 fluid ounces) Plain Yogurt (Whole Milk)
• 2 1/2 ounces Pineapple

- 20 each wholes Blanched & Slivered almonds
- 1/2 cup pure almond milk - unsweetened original

DIRECTIONS

Feel free to substitute other fruits or nuts for the pineapple and/or almonds (about 20 whole almonds, 3 Tbsp slivered). Be sure to use fresh pineapple in this smoothie. Canned pineapple is swimming in sugar.

Combine the yogurt, pineapple, almonds and almond milk in a blender and purée until smooth and creamy.

COOKING TIP: Whether you're feeding a family or cooking for one, you can update the serving settings above to reveal the required amount of ingredients.

Belgian Waffles Recipe
Prep Time: 10 Minutes
Style:French
Cook Time: 10 Minutes
Phase: Phase 1
Difficulty: Moderate

* Any adjustments made to the serving values will only update the ingredients of that recipe and not change the directions.
7.5g Protein, 7.6g Fat 1.7g Fiber, 115.9kcalCalories, Net Carbs 3.7g.

INGREDIENTS
• 1 cup whole grain soy flour
• 2 tablespoons sucralose based sweetener (Sugar Substitute)
• 3 teaspoons baking powder (Sodium Aluminum Sulfate, Double Acting)
• 1/2 teaspoon salt
• 1/4 cup heavy cream
• 3 large eggs
• 1 tablespoon sugar free syrup
• 1/4 cup (8 fluid ounces) water

DIRECTIONS
1. Heat waffle iron. Whisk together soy flour, sugar substitute, baking powder and salt. Add cream, eggs and syrup and stir

until well blended (batter will be stiff). Add cold water 1 tablespoon at a time until batter is easily spoonable and spreadable, about the consistency of a thick pancake batter.

2. Spray waffle iron with oil spray. Place approximately 3 tablespoons of batter in center of a waffle iron. Cook according to manufacturer's instructions until crisp and dark golden brown. Repeat with remaining batter. Serve warm.

COOKING TIP: Whether you're feeding a family or cooking for one, you can update the serving settings above to reveal the required amount of ingredients.

Bell Pepper Rings Filled with Eggs and Mozzarella Recipe

Prep Time: 10 Minutes
Style:American
Cook Time: 10 Minutes
Phase: Phase 1
Difficulty: Easy

* Any adjustments made to the serving values will only update the ingredients of that recipe and not change the directions.
19.6g Protein, 20.9g Fat 1.6g Fiber 292.1kcalCalories, Net Carbs 4.7g .

INGREDIENTS
• 1/2 large (approx 3-3/4" long, 3" dia) Bell Peppers
• 2 large Eggs (Whole)
• 1 teaspoon Canola Vegetable Oil
• 1/4 cup shredded Mozzarella Cheese (Whole Milk)

DIRECTIONS
1. Cut bell pepper in half across the middle, then cut two 1-inch rings. Remove seeds and ribs. Note that any color bell pepper works well in this recipe.
2. Place rings in sauté pan with oil over medium-high heat. Place an egg in each ring and cook until desired doneness (do not flip).
3. Top eggs with cheese and, cover pan and cook 1 more minute until cheese has melted. Season to taste with salt and freshly ground black pepper.
4. Serve immediately

COOKING TIP: Whether you're feeding a family or cooking for one, you can update the serving settings above to reveal the required amount of ingredients.

Berry Delicious Protein Shake Smoothie

Prep Time: 10 Minutes
Style:American
Cook Time: 0 Minutes
Phase: Phase 2
Difficulty: Easy

* Any adjustments made to the serving values will only update the ingredients of that recipe and not change the directions.
18.2g   Protein,   12.7g   Fat   13.8g
Fiber255.7kcalCalories, 7.5g Net Carbs.

INGREDIENTS
• 1 each Atkins Strawberry Shake
• 1 tablespoon Chia Seeds
• 1/2 cup Raspberries, fresh
• 1/4 cup Cucumber, raw, sliced
• 1/4 cup Kroger Riced Cauliflower, frozen (85g per 3/4 cup)

DIRECTIONS

For best results use a chilled Atkins shake.
Pour shake and chia seeds into a blender and let sit for 5 minutes. Add remaining ingredients and process until smooth.

Black Forest Protein Smoothie

Prep Time: 5 Minutes
Style:American
Cook Time: 0 Minutes
Phase: Phase 2
Difficulty: Easy

* Any adjustments made to the serving values will only update the ingredients of that recipe and not change the directions.
23.4g Protein, 5.7g Fat 2.6g Fiber 172.8kcalCalories, 6.7g Net Carbs.

INGREDIENTS

• 1/4 cup sweet cherries, frozen, unsweetened
• 1 cup coconut milk beverage, plain, unsweetened
• 1 scoop (1 scoop= 30 g) quest chocolate milkshake protein powder

DIRECTIONS

Blend all ingredients until very smooth. Pour over or blend with 1/2 cup of ice and enjoy.

Note that any sugar-free milk such as almond, soy or cashew may be substituted for the coconut.

COOKING TIP:Whether you're feeding a family or cooking for one, you can update the serving settings above to reveal the required amount of ingredients.

Blackberry Protein Smoothie Recipe

Prep Time: 5 Minutes
Style:American
Cook Time: 0 Minutes
Phase: Phase 2
Difficulty: Easy

* Any adjustments made to the serving values will only update the ingredients of that recipe and not change the directions.
16.5g Protein, 7.7g Fat, 8.1g Fiber 170.6kcalCalories, 7.2g Net Carbs.

INGREDIENTS
- 1/4 cup Blackberries, frozen, unsweetened
- 1 cup coconut milk beverage, plain, unsweetened
- 28 grams Atkins vanilla protein powder
- 1/8 teaspoon allspice, ground
- 1/8 teaspoon cinnamon, ground

DIRECTIONS
Blend all ingredients until very smooth. Pour over or blend with 1/2 cup of ice and enjoy.

Note that any sugar-free milk such as almond, soy or cashew may be sustituted for the coconut.

*28g = 1 scoop of Atkins Vanilla Protein Powder.

COOKING TIP: Whether you're feeding a family or cooking for one, you can update the serving settings above to reveal the required amount of ingredients.

Blackberry Smoothie Recipe

Prep Time: 5 Minutes
Style:American
Cook Time: 0 Minutes
Phase: Phase 2
Difficulty: Easy

* Any adjustments made to the serving values will only update the ingredients of that recipe and not change the directions.
25.3g Protein, 6.9g Fat, 5.2g Fiber, 209.7kcalCalories,6.4g Net Carbs.

INGREDIENTS
• 1/4 cup frozen blackberries
• 1 cup coconut milk unsweetened
• 1 ounce vanilla whey protein
• 1 tablespoon organic 100% whole ground Golden flaxseed meal
• 1/4 teaspoon cinnamon
• 1/16 teaspoon allspice ground
• 1/2 teaspoon vanilla extract

DIRECTIONS
For this recipe unsweetened coconut, almond or soy milk may be used. Combine the frozen balckberries, milk of choice,

protein powder, flax meal, vanilla and spices in a blender. Blend until smooth.

COOKING TIP: To make a colder smoothie, try adding a couple ice cubes to the mix before blending!

Blueberry Scones Recipe

Prep Time: 15 Minutes
Style:French
Cook Time: 55 Minutes
Phase: Phase 2
Difficulty: Moderate

* Any adjustments made to the serving values will only update the ingredients of that recipe and not change the directions.
7.3g Protein, 18.2g Fat, 2.2g Fiber, 218.5kcalCalories, 6.3g Net Carbs.

INGREDIENTS
• 1 1/2 cups whole grain soy flour
• 3 tablespoons sucralose based sweetener (sugar substitute)
• 1 teaspoon salt
• 3 teaspoons baking powder (sodium aluminum sulfate, double acting)

- 6 tablespoons unsalted butter stick
- 2/3 cup heavy cream
- 1/4 cup sour cream
- 1 large egg
- 1 cup blueberries
- 2 teaspoons lemon zest

DIRECTIONS

1. In a food processor, pulse soy flour, sugar substitute, salt, and baking powder for 5 seconds, just to combine. Add butter and pulse until mixture resembles a coarse meal, about 30 seconds.

2. Pour into a large mixing bowl and toss with blueberries and lemon zest. In a large liquid measuring cup or small bowl, whisk heavy cream, sour cream and egg until well-mixed.

3. Chill the dough for 30 minutes. Preheat oven to 375°F. Separate dough into 10 equal-sized balls and pat each piece into a disk measuring 2 to 3 across. Space disks evenly on an ungreased baking sheet, leaving one inch between each scone.

4. Bake scones until bottoms are golden brown and tops are light golden. Cool on baking sheet set on a wire rack.

COOKING TIP: We love the idea of customizing this recipe to make it your own! If you add any ingredients, just be sure to keep an eye on net carbs.

Breakfast Mexi Peppers Recipe

Prep Time: 30 Minutes
Style:American
Cook Time: 30 Minutes
Phase: Phase 1
Difficulty: Moderate

* Any adjustments made to the serving values will only update the ingredients of that recipe and not change the directions.
18.9g Protein, 22.7g Fat, 1.5g Fiber 307.6kcalCalories, 5g Net Carbs.

INGREDIENTS
• 4 ounces pork and beef chorizo
• 4 ounces ground beef (80% Lean / 20% Fat)
• 1/2 cup chopped onions
• 1/4 cup shredded cheddar cheese
• 3 large eggs (Whole)
• 2 medium (approx 2-3/4" long, 2-1/2" diameter) sweet red peppers

DIRECTIONS

1. Preheat oven to 400°F. Line a baking sheet with foil.

2. Cook chorizo, stirring to break up lumps, until browned. Drain excess fat.

3. Place chorizo and ground beef in mixing bowl and combine with the onion, cheese and eggs.

4. Cut peppers in half lengthwise. Scoop out seeds and cut away ribs.

5. Fill each pepper with one-quarter of the meat mixture. Place on the prepared baking sheet. Bake for 25-30 minutes and serve hot.

COOKING TIP: Whether you're feeding a family or cooking for one, you can update the serving settings above to reveal the required amount of ingredients.

Breakfast Burrito recipe

Prep Time: 15 Minutes
Style:Mexican
Cook Time: 5 Minutes
Phase: Phase 2
Difficulty: Moderate

* Any adjustments made to the serving values will only update the ingredients of that recipe and not change the directions.
18.4g Protein, 20.1g Fat, 5.1g Fiber 287.5kcalCalories, 6.5g Net Carbs.

INGREDIENTS
• 4 large eggs (Whole)
• 1/2 teaspoon salt
• 1/4 teaspoon ror cayenne pepper
• 2 tortillas low carb tortillas
• 1 tablespoon canola vegetable oil
• 3 tablespoons sweet red peppers
• 2 tablespoons chopped ccallions or spring Onions
• 1 Jalapeno pepper
• 1/8 teaspoon tabasco sauce
• 2 ounces sauce

DIRECTIONS

1. Whisk eggs, salt and cayenne together in a bowl.

2. In a medium skillet over medium heat, toast tortillas 1 minute per side until brown in spots; set aside and cover with foil to keep warm. Dice the red pepper, scallions (separate the white from the green parts) and finely dice the jalapeno.

3. In the same skillet add oil, red pepper, scallion whites and jalapeno. Cook until vegetables are softened, about 3 minutes.

4. Add eggs and continue to cook, stirring, until eggs are set, about 2 minutes.

5. Place tortillas on plates. Divide eggs between tortillas, season with hot sauce and gently roll up.

6. Serve with salsa and scallion greens.

Note: This can be made with a whole wheat or low-carb tortilla if you are in an acceptable phase. The whole wheat tortillas used here have 20g NC each so be sure to adjust the NC to the tortilla you are using. Low-carb tortillas typically have less NC than the whole wheat.

COOKING TIP: Whether you're feeding a family or cooking for one, you can update the serving settings above to reveal the required amount of ingredients.

Breakfast Berry Parfait Recipe

Prep Time: 15 Minutes
Style:American
Cook Time: 0 Minutes
Phase: Phase 2
Difficulty: Moderate

* Any adjustments made to the serving values will only update the ingredients of that recipe and not change the directions.
10.3g Protein, 25.3g Fat, 7.6g Fiber, 339.6kcalCalories, 11g Net Carbs.

INGREDIENTS
• 1 1/2 cup, wholes strawberries
• 2 cups raspberries
• 2 1/2 tablespoons sucralose based sweetener (sugar substitute)
• 1 cup heavy cream
• 1 tablespoon vanilla extract
• 6 ounces greek yogurt - plain (container)

- 1 each Atkins almond coconut bar

DIRECTIONS

1. In a blender, purée 1 1/2 cups of the strawberries and 1 1/2 cups of the raspberries with 1 1/2 tablespoons sugar substitute. Chop the remaining 1/2 cup raspberries and fold into the puree.

2. In a large mixing bowl, with an electric mixer on medium speed, combine heavy cream, the remaining 1 tablespoon sugar substitute and the vanilla, beating to soft peaks. Add yogurt (1 1/2 single-serving containers) and beat to stiff peaks.

3. In four parfait glasses, alternate layers of the berry mixture, cream filling and crumbled Atkins bar, making at least two layers of each.

4. Top each with some of the remaining 1/2 cup strawberries and serve.

COOKING TIP: Whether you're feeding a family or cooking for one, you can update the serving settings above to reveal the required amount of ingredients.

Blueberry, Maple and Pecan Smoothie Recipe
Prep Time: 5 Minutes
Style:American
Cook Time: 0 Minutes
Phase: Phase 2
Difficulty: Easy

* Any adjustments made to the serving values will only update the ingredients of that recipe and not change the directions.
26.6g Protein, 15.3g Fat, 3.3g Fiber, 281.8kcalCalories, 9.6g Net Carbs.

INGREDIENTS
• 1/4 cup blueberries, fresh
• 10 each pecan Halves, raw
• 1 cup coconut milk beverage, plain, unsweetened
• 1 scoop (1 scoop= 31 g) quest vanilla milkshake protein powder
• 1 tablespoon maple syrup (sugar-free)
• 1 tablespoon lemon juice

DIRECTIONS

Blend all ingredients except ice until very smooth. Pour over or blend with 1/2 cup of ice and enjoy.

Note that any sugar-free milk such as almond, soy or cashew may be sustituted for the coconut.

COOKING TIP: Why not have friends over to enjoy this drink! Update the serving settings above to reveal the required amount of ingredients you'll need.

Breakfast Sausage Sautéed with Red and Green Bell Peppers Recipe

Prep Time: 5 Minutes
Style:Other
Cook Time: 10 Minutes
Phase: Phase 1
Difficulty: Easy

* Any adjustments made to the serving values will only update the ingredients of that recipe and not change the directions.
29.8g Protein, 20.9g Fat, 1.5g Fiber, 328.4kcalCalories, 3.1g Net Carbs.

INGREDIENTS

- 1 teaspoon canola vegetable oil
- 4 link, cookeds turkey breakfast sausage
- 1/4 large (2.25 per pound, approx 3-3/4" long, 3" diameter) red sweet pepper
- 1/4 large (2.25 per pound, approx 3-3/4" long, 3" diameter) green sweet pepper
- 1 slice (1 ounce) monterey jack cheese

DIRECTIONS

1. Heat a skillet with 1 teaspoon oil over medium-high heat.

2. Crumble the sausage link or leave whole and slice after cooking. Sauté until just beginning to brown. About 3 minutes. Dice the peppers and add them to the sausage. Cook until sausage is browned and peppers are softened, about 5 minutes.

3. Sprinkle cheese on top and allow to melt 1-2 minutes. Serve immediately.

COOKING TIP: Whether you're feeding a family or cooking for one, you can update the serving settings above to reveal the required amount of ingredients.

Broccolini and Bacon Egg Bites Recipe

Prep Time: 5 Minutes
Style:American
Cook Time: 40 Minutes
Phase: Phase 1
Difficulty: Moderate

* Any adjustments made to the serving values will only update the ingredients of that recipe and not change the directions.
14.8g Protein, 23.1g Fat, 0.3g Fiber, 282.6kcalCalories, 3.4g Net Carbs.

 INGREDIENTS
• 8 servings olive oil palm (0.5g = 0.6sec spray)
• 5 slices bacon
• 6 stalks broccolini, fresh, steamed
• 5 each egg
• 6 tablespoons cream cheese, original
• 1 ounce feta cheese
• 3 teaspoons hot sauce - cholula hot sauce
• 1/2 teaspoon(s) kosher salt (1/4 tsp= 1.5 g)
• 1 1/2 cups arugula, raw
• 1 tablespoon lemon juice
• 1 tablespoon olive oil
• 1/8 teaspoon black pepper, ground

DIRECTIONS

Preheat the oven to 350°F. Lightly coat eight silicone egg-bite mold cups or eight cups of a standard nonstick muffin tin with cooking spray, or line a regular (not nonstick) muffin tin with nonstick muffin liners and set into a large baking pan.

In a large nonstick skillet, cook the bacon over medium heat until golden, about 5 minutes per side. Transfer to a paper towel-lined plate to drain. Chop the bacon into small pieces.

Meanwhile, in a blender, puree the eggs, cream cheese, feta cheese, hot sauce, and 1/4 teaspoon salt until smooth.

Pour off all but 1 tablespoon of fat from the skillet. Add the broccolini, 1 tablespoon water, and 1/4 teaspoon salt. Cook over medium-high heat, stirring frequently, until the broccolini is tender, 3 to 5 minutes. Remove from the heat.

Fill each of the egg cups with 1 heaping teaspoon of bacon and one heaping tablespoon of broccolini. Top with the egg mixture, filling the cups to about 1 inch from the top (you may have a bit left over; discard or saute in a skillet for a mini snack). Add just enough boiled water to the baking pan to come halfway up the sides of the molds.

Bake the egg bites until set, 20 to 25 minutes. Take the pan from the oven, then take the molds from the water bath. Let the egg bites cool for a few minutes, then take them from the molds.

In a medium bowl, toss together the arugula, lemon juice, oil, and a pinch each of salt and pepper. Place 3/4 cup of salad and 2 egg bites on each of four plates and serve.

Adapt this recipe for Atkins 40 by adding 1/4 cup fresh blueberries per serving
Adapt this recipe for Atkins 100 by adding 1 slice toasted Ezekiel sprouted grain bread per serving

COOKING TIP: This and 50 other delicious and adaptable recipes can be found in The Atkins 100 Eating Solution, Easy Low-Carb Living for Everyday Wellness

LOW CARB DINNER & ENTRÉE RECIPES

Nachos Stuffed Chicken Breast Recipe

Prep Time: 25 Minutes
Style:Mexican
Cook Time: 25 Minutes
Phase: Phase 1
Difficulty: Moderate

* Any adjustments made to the serving values will only update the ingredients of that recipe and not change the directions.
79.5g Protein, 31.6g Fat, 1.8g Fiber, 650.1kcalCalories, 6.8g Net Carbs.

INGREDIENTS
• 4 ounces cabot pepper jack cheese
• 1/3 cup sour cream
• 1 medium (4-1/8" long) scallions, raw
• 2 tablespoons cilantro, fresh, chopped
• 1 3/4 teaspoon(s) Kosher salt (1/4 tsp= 1.5 g)
• 32 ounces chicken breast filet, skinless

- 2 teaspoons chili powder
- 2 servings olive oil pam (0.5g = 0.6sec spray)
- 1 each tomato, medium 4.6 oz
- 4 tablespoons lime juice
- 3 tablespoons olive oil
- 1/2 teaspoon erythritol
- 1/8 teaspoon black pepper, ground
- 5 cup (47.3g) mixed baby greens

DIRECTIONS

Preheat the oven to 400°F.

In a small bowl, combine the cheese, sour cream, scallion, cilantro, and 1/2 teaspoon salt.

Insert a small sharp knife into the thickest part of each chicken breast and push it three-quarters of the way down to the thin end, being careful not to pierce the outside of the breast. Move the knife from side to side to form a wide pocket with a opening.

Stuff each breast with a quarter of the cheese mixture (about 1/4 cup). Secure with toothpicks. Season the chicken with the chili powder and 1 teaspoon salt.

Lightly coat a large ovenproof skillet with cooking spray and heat over medium-high heat until hot but not smoking. Place the chicken breasts into the skillet and cook until golden, about 2 minutes per side. Transfer the skillet to the oven and roast until an instant-read thermometer inserted into the thickest part of the breast reads 165°F, 18 to 20 minutes.

Meanwhile, prepare the dressing: in a small bowl, whisk the lime juice, oil, erythritol, and a generous pinch each of salt and pepper together until combined.

Remove the chicken from the oven. Remove and discard the toothpicks, then arrange the chicken on four serving plates. Mound 1 1/4 cups greens alongside each chicken breast, then drizzle the greens with about 1 1/2 tablespoons of dressing per serving. Top each portion with 2 heaping tablespoons of chopped tomato and cilantro to taste and serve.

Adapt for Atkins 40 by serving with 2 tablespoons canned refried black beans per serving
Adapt for Atkins 100 by serving with ½ cup canned refried black beans per serving

COOKING TIP: This and 50 other delicious and adaptable recipes can be found in The Atkins 100 Eating Solution, Easy Low-Carb Living for Everyday Wellness.

Acorn Squash with Spiced Applesauce and Maple Drizzle Recipe

Prep Time: 8 Minutes
Style:American
Cook Time: 20 Minutes
Phase: Phase 3
Difficulty: Moderate

* Any adjustments made to the serving values will only update the ingredients of that recipe and not change the directions.
0.7g Protein, 3.3g Fat, 2.2g Fiber, 72.8kcalCalories, 9.7g Net Carbs.

INGREDIENTS
• 1 squash (4 inch diameter) acorn winter squash
• 5 teaspoons unsalted butter stick
• 1/2 teaspoon salt
• 1/2 teaspoon black pepper
• 3/4 cup applesauce (without added ascorbic acid, unsweetened, canned)
• 1/8 teaspoon cinnamon
• 1 tablespoon sugar free maple flavored syrup

DIRECTIONS

1. Preheat oven to 350°F. Cut squash in half, remove seeds and then cut into 6 wedges.

2. Line a sheet pan with aluminum foil. Melt 1 tablespoon (3 teaspoons) butter and brush on squash; sprinkle with salt and pepper. Place on pan and bake until squash is fork tender, about 20 minutes.

3. In a small pot heat the applesauce, about 3 minutes. Stir in 2 teaspoons butter and cinnamon and cook 30 seconds more.

4. Serve squash with a dollop of applesauce mixture and a drizzle of syrup (about 1/2 teaspoon each).

COOKING TIP: Having a party? When planning your low carb spread, think about which dishes you can make in advance and which need fresh ingredients that day.

Air-Fryer One Pot Chicken and Vegetables
Prep Time: 10 Minutes
Style:American
Cook Time: 25 Minutes
Phase: Phase 4
Difficulty: Easy

* Any adjustments made to the serving values will only update the ingredients of that recipe and not change the directions.
46.1g Protein, 45.5g Fat, 6.2g Fiber, 709.6kcalCalories, Net Carbs 20.8g.

INGREDIENTS
• 6 ounces chicken thigh, boneless, with skin
• 1/2 sweetpotato, 5" long sweet potato
• 4 teaspoons ghee
• 1/4 teaspoon Salt
• 1/4 teaspoon Black Pepper, ground
• 1 cup Red Cabbage, steamed, shredded
• 1/8 tablespoon apple cider vinegar
• 1/8 teaspoon cayenne pepper
• 1/16 teaspoon (3.5g) truvia
• 1/16 teaspoon Chili powder
• 1/16 teaspoon garlic powder
• 1/16 teaspoon paprika

DIRECTIONS

1. Preheat air fryer to 375°F for at least 3 minutes. Season both sides of the chicken thigh with salt and pepper, and cook skin side down in the air fryer alone for 12 minutes.

2. While the chicken begins to cook, cut the sweet potato into ½-inch julienne, or French fry shape. Toss with 1 tablespoon melted ghee, 1/8 teaspoon salt and 1/8 teaspoon pepper.

3. When the chicken has reached the 12 minute mark, turn it over and add the sweet potato fries to the air fryer in a single layer. Continue to cook for 5 minutes.

4. While the sweet potatoes and chicken cook, slice two 1-inch thick "steaks" from the cabbage. Spread each side of each cabbage slice with ½ teaspoon ghee and season with a pinch of salt and pepper. After 5 minutes of cooking the sweet potatoes and chicken, shake the fryer basket to toss the sweet potatoes, and add the cabbage on top of the chicken and sweet potatoes. Cook all the components for another 8 minutes.

5. While the cooking completes, combine the vinegar with 1 teaspoon ghee, cayenne,

stevia and erythritol sweetener, chili powder, garlic, and paprika in a small bowl. This recipe gives a medium level of spice. If you prefer your chicken more spicy, you can double the amount of cayenne.

6. Remove the cabbage and sweet potatoes from the air fryer to a plate. Check the chicken for doneness using an instant read thermometer to ensure an internal temperature of 165°. Remove the fully cooked chicken from the air fryer and spread each side of the chicken with half of the spicy oil.

Keto Alfredo Sauce Recipe

Prep Time: 20 Minutes
Style:Italian
Cook Time: 0 Minutes
Phase: Phase 1
Difficulty: Easy

* Any adjustments made to the serving values will only update the ingredients of that recipe and not change the directions.
10.5g Protein, 33.3g Fat, 0g Fiber, 348.6kcalCalories, 2.7g Net Carbs.

INGREDIENTS
- 2 tablespoons unsalted butter stick
- 1 1/2 cups heavy cream
- 1/2 cup parmesan cheese (trated)
- 4 ounces romano cheese
- 1/8 teaspoon black pepper
- 1/8 teaspoon nutmeg (Ground)

DIRECTIONS
One of the simplest and best of all pasta sauces, Alfredo sauce is versatile enough to dress up steamed vegetables as well. For the best flavor, buy blocks of Parmesan and Pecorino Romano and grate them yourself. See a variation below. Each serving is 1/4 cup.

1. Melt butter in a medium saucepan over medium heat. Add cream and simmer until reduced to 1 cup, about 10 minutes. Grate Parmesan and Romano cheeses.
2. Remove from heat; stir in Parmesan, Romano, pepper and nutmeg until the cheeses have melted and sauce is smooth.
3. Serve immediately.
Vodka Sauce: Prepare Alfredo Sauce according   to   directions,   adding   3

tablespoons tomato paste and 2 tablespoons vodka to the heavy cream before reducing.

COOKING TIP: Alfredo sauce on zoodles are delish! Try our Zucchini Chicken Alfredo recipe.

Nachos Stuffed Chicken Breast Recipe

Prep Time: 25 Minutes
Style:Mexican
Cook Time: 25 Minutes
Phase: Phase 1
Difficulty: Moderate

* Any adjustments made to the serving values will only update the ingredients of that recipe and not change the directions.
79.5g Protein, 31.6g Fat, 1.8g Fiber, 650.1kcalCalories, 6.8g Net Carbs.

INGREDIENTS
• 4 ounces cabot pepper jack cheese
• 1/3 cup sour cream
• 1 medium (4-1/8" long) scallions, raw
• 2 tablespoons Cilantro, fresh, chopped
• 1 3/4 teaspoon(s) Kosher salt (1/4 tsp= 1.5 g)

- 32 ounces chicken breast filet, skinless
- 2 teaspoons chili powder
- 2 servings olive oil Pam (0.5g = 0.6sec spray)
- 1 each Tomato, medium 4.6 oz
- 4 tablespoons lime juice
- 3 tablespoons olive oil
- 1/2 teaspoon erythritol
- 1/8 teaspoon black pepper, ground
- 5 cup (47.3g) mixed baby greens

DIRECTIONS

Preheat the oven to 400°F.

In a small bowl, combine the cheese, sour cream, scallion, cilantro, and 1/2 teaspoon salt.

Insert a small sharp knife into the thickest part of each chicken breast and push it three-quarters of the way down to the thin end, being careful not to pierce the outside of the breast. Move the knife from side to side to form a wide pocket with a opening. Stuff each breast with a quarter of the cheese mixture (about 1/4 cup). Secure with toothpicks. Season the chicken with the chili powder and 1 teaspoon salt.

Lightly coat a large ovenproof skillet with cooking spray and heat over medium-high heat until hot but not smoking. Place the chicken breasts into the skillet and cook until golden, about 2 minutes per side. Transfer the skillet to the oven and roast until an instant-read thermometer inserted into the thickest part of the breast reads 165°F, 18 to 20 minutes.

Meanwhile, prepare the dressing: in a small bowl, whisk the lime juice, oil, erythritol, and a generous pinch each of salt and pepper together until combined.

Remove the chicken from the oven. Remove and discard the toothpicks, then arrange the chicken on four serving plates. Mound 1 1/4 cups greens alongside each chicken breast, then drizzle the greens with about 1 1/2 tablespoons of dressing per serving. Top each portion with 2 heaping tablespoons of chopped tomato and cilantro to taste and serve.

Adapt for Atkins 40 by serving with 2 tablespoons canned refried black beans per serving

Adapt for Atkins 100 by serving with ½ cup canned refried black beans per serving

COOKING TIP: This and 50 other delicious and adaptable recipes can be found in The

Atkins 100 Eating Solution, Easy Low-Carb Living for Everyday Wellness.

LOW CARB SNACK RECIPES

Keto Air Fryer Jalapeno Poppers

Prep Time: 20 Minutes
Style:American
Cook Time: 15 Minutes
Phase: Phase 1
Difficulty: Easy

* Any adjustments made to the serving values will only update the ingredients of that recipe and not change the directions.
3.3g Protein, 5.9g Fat, 0.6g Fiber, 71.7kcalCalories, 1.1g Net Carbs-

INGREDIENTS
• 7 tablespoons cream cheese, original
• 1/4 cup shredded cheddar cheese
• 1/4 cup shredded monterey cheese
• 1/2 teaspoon chili powder
• 240 Jalapeno peppers
• 6 slices bacon

Ingredient note: 240 grams of jalapenos is equivalent to 6 (3-4-inch) jalapenos.

DIRECTIONS

1. Heat air fryer to 390°F.

2. In a small bowl, combine the cream cheese, cheddar, Monterey jack, and chili powder until well combined and evenly distributed.

3. Slice each jalapeno in half lengthwise. Use a spoon to scoop out the seeds and discard, then fill with cream cheese mix (do not overfill). Slice the bacon in half, and loosely drape a slice of bacon over each filled jalapeno, securing the bacon on the top and bottom with a toothpick or skewer.

4. Cook, in batches if needed, for 6 minutes, or until the bacon is crispy and the cheese has melted. Remove from air fryer and serve.

COOKING TIP: This naturally keto and low carb recipe is a great for sharing!

Asian Chicken Handrolls with Peanut Sauce Recipe

Prep Time: 0 Minutes
Style:Asian
Cook Time: 0 Minutes
Phase: Phase 2
Difficulty: Difficult

* Any adjustments made to the serving values will only update the ingredients of that recipe and not change the directions.
33.9g Protein, 23.9g Fat, 7.3g Fiber, 414kcalCalories, 8.3g Net Carbs.

 INGREDIENTS
• 8 ounces chicken yenderloins
• 1 1/2 tablespoons organic tamari
• 1 tablespoon rice vinegar
• 1 teaspoon ginger
• 1 serving liquid Stevia
• 1/2 avocado, florida or californium Avocados
• 1/4 cucumber (8-1/4") Cucumber (with Peel)
• 2 1/2 ounces yambean (Jicama)
• 8 sprigs cilantro
• 2 sheets sushi nori roasted seaweed
• 1/2 tablespoon vegetable oil

- 1 1/2 servings 100% natural creamy Peanut Butter
- 4 tablespoons tap water
- 3/4 teaspoon sriracha chili sauce

DIRECTIONS

1. Marinate the chicken tenderloins by placing them in a plastic bag with 1 tbsp tamari, 1 tbsp rice vinegar, 1/2 tsp minced ginger and 3-4 drops stevia. Set aside.

2. While the chicken marinates prepare the vegetables. Slice the avocado into 8 long pieces. Cut the cucumber and jicama into sticks measuring about 3 x 1/8 inches. Divide ingredients into 4 equal sets. Set all aside on a cutting board along with the sprigs of cilantro. Gently fold the nori sheets in half and then rip them in two, set all 4 sheets aside.

3. Place the vegetable oil in a nonstick skillet over medium-high heat. Add the chicken, discarding the remaining marinade and plastic bag. Cook until no longer pink in the center; about 3 minutes per side. Place on the cutting board with the other ingredients and slice each tenderloin into 3 pieces (if you only had 3 tenderloins, cut into an amount that is easily divided by 4).

Place a small dish of water next to the assembly line. Set aside.

4. In a small bowl combine the peanut butter, water, 1 1/2 tsp tamari, 1/2 tsp minced ginger, 3-4 drops stevia and 3/4 tsp sriracha. Blend until all ingredients are incorporated, adjust seasonings to your taste by adding more tamari, ginger, stevia or sriracha.

5. Assembly: Place the 1/2 sheet of nori on a flat surface. Place the sliced avocado, cucumber, jicama, and cilantro at a slight angle so they align with the corner of one end of the nori sheet with about 1/2-inch of the corner of the nori sheet sticking out. Dredge the chicken in the peanut sauce and place it on top of the vegetables. Roll, starting at the side where you placed the ingredients, then change direction slightly so that it creates a cone shape with one end rolling tightly and the other end open. With your finger tips, dip them in the water bowl, and add water to the nori sheet on the end corner of the wrap, hold it down a few seconds to seal the wrap in place. Repeat for remaining wraps.

6. Serve wraps with any remaining sauce for dipping.

COOKING TIP: Whether you're feeding a family or cooking for one, you can update the serving settings above to reveal the required amount of ingredients.

Air Fryer Korean Chicken Wings

Prep Time: 250 Minutes
Style:Asian
Cook Time: 30 Minutes
Phase: Phase 1
Difficulty: Easy

* Any adjustments made to the serving values will only update the ingredients of that recipe and not change the directions.
17.7g Protein, 21.5g Fat, 1.4g Fiber, 291.5kcalCalories, 1.7g Net Carbs.

INGREDIENTS
• 1/2 cup kimchi kraut juice
• 1 cup buttermilk, whole milk
• 4 tablespoons sambal oelek ground fresh Chili Paste
• 1 each egg
• 2 each garlic, clove
• 1 teaspoon salt
• 1 teaspoon black pepper, ground

- 2 pounds chicken wing, meat and skin, raw
- 1/2 cup kimchi, cabbage
- 8 tablespoons mayonnaise (Hellman's Real)
- 6 teaspoons sriracha hot sauce (Rooster sauce)

DIRECTIONS

1. Using a fine mesh strainer collect ½ cup juice from the kimchi. Use a clean kitchen towel and squeeze the kimchi to release more juice if needed. Mince or press the garlic. In a small bowl, use a fork to whisk together the kimchi juice, buttermilk, red chili paste, egg, garlic, salt, and pepper.

2. Place the chicken wings in a zipper-lock freezer bag, pour in the buttermilk mixture, and toss to coat. Place in the refrigerator to marinate for at least 4 hours or overnight, turning at least a few times to ensure even coating with the marinade.

3. Preheat your air fryer to 390°F for about 10 minutes.

4. Place the chicken in a single layer in the warm Air Fryer and cook for 9-10 minutes for drumettes, 7-8 minutes for wings, or until chicken reaches an internal temperature of 165°F, turning once in the middle of the

cooking time. Complete this step in batches if needed.

5. In a food processor, chop the strained and squeezed out kimchi until it is fine pieces. Add the mayonnaise and Sriracha and process until it is the consistency of tartar sauce. Serve alongside the chicken wings as a dipping sauce. One serving is about 2 wings and 1 ½ tablespoons dipping sauce.

NOTE: Because only about about 30% of the marinade is likely to be consumed, corrected nutritionals per serving for this recipe are as follows: Total carbs- 2.15; Net carbs- 1.67; Protein- 16.44; Fiber- 0.48; Fat- 20.18; Calories- 260.9

Air Fryer Pepperoni Chips Recip

Prep Time: 0 Minutes
Style:Italian
Cook Time: 4 Minutes
Phase: Phase 1
Difficulty: Easy

* Any adjustments made to the serving values will only update the ingredients of that recipe and not change the directions. 5.7g Protein, 11.3g Fat, 0.4g Fiber, 130.5kcalCalories, 0.7g Net Carbs.

INGREDIENTS
• 56 grams Pepperoni
Ingredient Notes: We used 3-inch diameter pepperoni slices that are ¼-ounce each. Changing the size and thickness of the pepperoni will change the optimal cooking time.

DIRECTIONS
1. Preheat your air fryer to 390°F for at least 3 minutes.
2. Create a single layer with only minimal overlap of pepperoni on the fryer plate. Cover with the dehydrator rack to help keep

the pepperoni in place. Fry for 3 minutes 30 seconds.

3. Remove pepperoni slices from the air fryer and allow to cool on a paper towel lined plate for at least 1 minute. Repeat steps 2 and 3 if needed to fry all the pepperoni slices.

4. These chips can be eaten as is, or dipped in guacamole for a delicious snack!

Apple Muffins with Cinnamon-Pecan Streusel Recipe

Prep Time: 15 Minutes
Style:American
Cook Time: 25 Minutes
Phase: Phase 3
Difficulty: Moderate

* Any adjustments made to the serving values will only update the ingredients of that recipe and not change the directions.

7.6g Protein, 21.1g Fat, 5.1g Fiber, 246.6kcalCalories, 5.2g Net Carbs.

INGREDIENTS
- 1 2/3 cups almond meal flour
- 1/2 cup, half pecans
- 6 1/2 teaspoons cinnamon
- 1/3 teaspoon salt
- 6 tablespoons erythritol
- 1/16 pinch stevia
- 2 tablespoons unsalted butter stick
- 2 large eggs (Whole)
- 1/4 cup coconut milk unsweetened
- 2 teaspoons vanilla extract
- 2 tablespoons organic high fiber coconut Flour
- 1 teaspoon baking powder (Straight Phosphate, Double Acting)
- 2/3 cup, quartered or chopped apple

DIRECTIONS

1. Preheat oven to 350 F. Prepare a muffin tin with 8 cupcake papers.

2. Combine 2/3 cup almond flour, chopped pecans, 2 tablespoons cinnamon, 1/8 teaspoon salt, 2 tablespoons granular sugar substitute (eryhtritol), a pinch of stevia and 2 tablespoons melted butter in a small bowl. Mix with a fork until it begins to crumble. Set aside while making the muffin batter.

3. For the muffins: whisk together the eggs, 1/4 cup coconut milk, 2 teaspoons vanilla, 6

tablespoons granular sugar substitute (erythritol), a pinch of stevia, and 1/2 teaspoon ground cinnamon. Add 1 cup almond flour, 2 tablespoons coconut flour, 1/4 teaspoon salt and 1 teaspoon baking powder; mix to combine then fold in 2/3 cup finely chopped apples.

4. Divide into muffin 8 wells topping each with about 2 tablespoons of the struesal. Bake for 25 minutes, remove from oven and allow to sit for 10-20 minutes to cool before removing. These may be eaten immediately or stored in an airtight container in the refrigerator for up to 1 week.

COOKING TIP: We love the idea of customizing this recipe to make it your own! If you add any ingredients, just be sure to keep an eye on net carbs.

Atkins Mini Muffins Recipe

Prep Time: 10 Minutes
Style:American
Cook Time: 25 Minutes
Phase: Phase 3
Difficulty: Moderate

* Any adjustments made to the serving
values will only update the ingredients of
that recipe and not change the directions.
5.6g Protein, 4.4g Fat, 0.8g Fiber,
71.5kcalCalories, 2.1g Net Carbs.

INGREDIENTS
• 3 teaspoons baking powder (Straight
Phosphate, Double Acting)
• 1/3 cup sucralose based sweetener (Sugar
Substitute)
• 2 tablespoons unsalted butter stick
• 1 cup sour cream (Cultured)
• 2 large eggs (Whole)
• 6 servings Atkins flour mix

DIRECTIONS

Use the Atkins recipe to make Atkins Flour Mix for this recipe, you will need 2 cups.

1. Preheat oven to 350°F.

2. Blend all dry ingredients together in a large mixing bowl. Then add wet ingredients with a spoon or spatula and mix thoroughly.

3. Lightly coat mini muffin tins with non-stick vegetable oil spray (or use paper mini muffin cups).

4. Spoon dough mixture into mini muffin tins and bake for 18-22 minutes or until done. Recipe makes 24 mini muffins. *Add berries if desired but remember to account for additional Net Carbs.

COOKING TIP: Whether you're feeding a family or cooking for one, you can update the serving settings above to reveal the required amount of ingredients.

Baked Goat Cheese and Ricotta Custards Recipe
Prep Time: 0 Minutes
Style:Italian
Cook Time: 50 Minutes
Phase: Phase 2
Difficulty: Moderate

* Any adjustments made to the serving values will only update the ingredients of that recipe and not change the directions.
22.4g Protein, 27.8g Fat, 1.1g Fiber, 356.6kcalCalories, 4.1g Net Carbs

INGREDIENTS
• 1 cup ricotta cheese (Whole Milk)
• 6 ounces goats cheese (Semisoft)
• 3 tablespoons parmesan cheese (Grated)
• 1/4 cup chopped english walnuts
• 2 tablespoons basil
• 2 large eggs (Whole)
• 1/8 teaspoon Salt
• 1/8 teaspoon black pepper
• 12 leaves spinach

DIRECTIONS

This recipe is suitable for all phases except the first two weeks of Induction due ot the nuts.

1. Heat oven to 350°F. Spray cooking spray onto four 5-ounce ramekins or custard cups.

2. Combine ricotta, goat cheese, Parmesan, walnuts, basil, egg, salt, and pepper in a bowl and mix well.

3. Line each ramekin with 3 spinach leaves. Divide cheese mixture; fill full. Bake 30 minutes. Cool 5 minutes.

4. To serve, run a knife around the rim of each custard. Invert onto small plates. Season with salt and pepper to taste.

Note: Photo shown includes Atkins Pie Crust which contains gluten and is not suitable until Phase 3. Follow link to recipe, make full recipe, rolling out just enough to fill mini muffin tins with the custard recipe above. Prebake the crusts for 8 min then fill and bake another 30 minutes. You will have some leftover crust - simply form into a disk and freeze for another use.

COOKING TIP: Having a party? When planning your low carb spread, think about which dishes you can make in advance and which need fresh ingredients that day.

LOW CARB APPETIZERS & SIDE DISH RECIPES

Artichokes with Lemon-Butter Recipe

Prep Time: 10 Minutes
Style:Other
Cook Time: 15 Minutes
Phase: Phase 1
Difficulty: Easy

* Any adjustments made to the serving values will only update the ingredients of that recipe and not change the directions.
5.4g Protein, 23.8g Fat 9.6g Fiber, 287.9kcalCalories, 10.7g Net Carbs.

INGREDIENTS
• 4 artichoke, media Artichokes (Globe or French)
• 4 fruit (2-1/8" diameter) Lemon
• 2 tablespoons coriander seed
• 2 tablespoons salt
• 1/2 cup unsalted butter stick

DIRECTIONS

1. Bring 4 quarts of water to a boil in a large pot. Trim the stems of the artichokes to about 2 inches.

2. Halve 3 lemons and squeeze juice into water. Add lemon halves, coriander seeds and salt. Place artichokes in the cooking liquid, and cover with a heavy plate to keep them from floating. Boil 15 minutes, until a paring knife, inserted where the stem meets the bottom, comes out easily. Remove and drain excess water.

3. In a small bowl, melt butter in a microwave or saucepan. Mix in juice of remaining lemon, salt and pepper.

4. Serve each person one whole artichoke, accompanied by a ramekin of butter sauce and a large bowl for discarded leaves. Season with freshly ground salt and pepper to taste.

COOKING TIP: Having a party? When planning your low carb spread, think about which dishes you can make in advance and which need fresh ingredients that day.

Acorn Squash with Spiced Applesauce and Maple Drizzle Recipe

Prep Time: 8 Minutes
Style:American
Cook Time: 20 Minutes
Phase: Phase 3
Difficulty: Moderate

* Any adjustments made to the serving values will only update the ingredients of that recipe and not change the directions.
0.7g Protein, 3.3g Fat, 2.2g Fiber, 72.8kcalCalories,9.7g Net Carbs.

INGREDIENTS
• 1 squash (4 inch diameter) Acorn Winter Squash
• 5 teaspoons unsalted butter stick
• 1/2 teaspoon salt
• 1/2 teaspoon Black Pepper
• 3/4 cup Applesauce (without added ascorbic acid, unsweetened, canned)
• 1/8 teaspoon Cinnamon
• 1 tablespoon Sugar free maple flavored Syrup

DIRECTIONS

1. Preheat oven to 350°F. Cut squash in half, remove seeds and then cut into 6 wedges.

2. Line a sheet pan with aluminum foil. Melt 1 tablespoon (3 teaspoons) butter and brush on squash; sprinkle with salt and pepper. Place on pan and bake until squash is fork tender, about 20 minutes.

3. In a small pot heat the applesauce, about 3 minutes. Stir in 2 teaspoons butter and cinnamon and cook 30 seconds more.

4. Serve squash with a dollop of applesauce mixture and a drizzle of syrup (about 1/2 teaspoon each).

COOKING TIP: Having a party? When planning your low carb spread, think about which dishes you can make in advance and which need fresh ingredients that day.

"Pasta" Salad with Pesto and Zucchini Ribbons Recipe

Prep Time: 10 Minutes
Style:Italian
Cook Time: 0 Minutes
Phase: Phase 2
Difficulty: Easy

* Any adjustments made to the serving values will only update the ingredients of that recipe and not change the directions.
4.2g Protein, 11.9g Fat, 1.8g Fiber, 150.6kcalCalories, 5.9g Net Carbs.

INGREDIENTS
• 2 cups zucchini noodles
• 10 each cherry or grape tomato
• 1/4 cup green bell pepper (chopped)
• 1/4 cup red bell pepper (chopped)
• 1/4 cup Red Onion (chopped)
• 16 each Kalamata Olives
• 1/4 cup, crumbled Feta Cheese
• 1 serving Basil Pesto
Ingredient notes: You will need ¼ cup of Atkins recipe for basil pesto, or you can use a premade pesto with no more than 2 net carbs for ¼ cup. We suggest using 2-inch long zucchini ribbons, or wavy ribbons, for

this recipe. Optionally, sprinkle with 2 tablespoons pine nuts for an extra 0.4 net carbs per serving.

DIRECTIONS
1. Fold together all ingredients in a medium bowl until evenly distributed and coated with pesto.

Kid friendly variation: Use 16 large black olives and 1-ounce mozzarella cheese instead of the Kalamata olives and feta cheese, and subtract 0.7 Net Carbs per serving.

Air Fryer Buffalo Cauliflower Recipe
Prep Time: 10 Minutes
Style:American
Cook Time: 5 Minutes
Phase: Phase 1
Difficulty: Moderate

* Any adjustments made to the serving values will only update the ingredients of that recipe and not change the directions.
32.3g Protein, 29.5g Fat, 2.6g Fiber, 419.4kcalCalories.

INGREDIENTS

- 5 servings Kroger Pork Rinds (1/2 ounce)
- 9 teaspoons Frank's Redhot Buffalo Wings Sauce
- 1 1/2 tablespoons Butter - Unsalted - Kroger Brand
- 2 1/4 servings Hot Sauce, Sriracha Hot Chili Sauce 1 teaspoon (5grams)
- 2/3 tablespoon Apple Cider Vinegar
- 1/4 head large (6-7" diameter) Cauliflower, raw
- 1 each Egg
- 1 1/2 ounces Maytag Blue Cheese

DIRECTIONS

1. Preheat your air fryer to 390°F for about 10 minutes while you are preparing the cauliflower.

2. Pulse 2.5 ounces of pork rinds in a food processor until they are broken down to a sand like texture, being careful not to over process into a paste. Measure out ¼ cup plus 2 tablespoons of the ground pork rinds into a large bowl. Add the hot wing sauce, melted butter, Sriracha, and vinegar to the pork rinds and stir until well combined. It will be a thick batter consistency.

3. In another medium to large bowl, whisk the egg until frothy.

4. Cut the cauliflower into florets, ensuring none are overly large, and place in the bowl with the egg. Toss to coat, ensuring that the egg gets into as many nooks and crannies in the cauliflower as possible. Then, one by one, coat each floret in the wing sauce batter, smoothing it onto the surface and into the nooks of the cauliflower so each floret is nicely coated.

5. Once the air fryer is preheated, arrange the cauliflower in a single layer in the basket. Cook for 5 minutes at 390°F. Remove from the fryer, sprinkle with the blue cheese and serve while hot.

Atkins Peanut Butter Granola Bar Parfait with Yogurt and Strawberries Recipe

Prep Time: 5 Minutes
Style:American
Cook Time: 0 Minutes
Phase: Phase 3
Difficulty: Easy

* Any adjustments made to the serving values will only update the ingredients of that recipe and not change the directions.
27.9g Protein, 11.3g Fat, 7.8g Fiber, 309.2kcalCalories, 13.6g Net Carbs.

INGREDIENTS
• 1/2 cup Greek Yogurt - Plain (Container)
• 5 large (1-3/8" diameter) Strawberries
• 1 each Atkins Peanut Butter Granola Bar

DIRECTIONS
This recipe uses one Atkins Peanut Butter Granola Bar that has been coarsely chopped. Another Atkins bar with 4g NC or less may be substituted as desired.

In a parfait glass, layer the chopped granola bar with the yogurt and diced or quartered strawberries.

COOKING TIP: Whether you're feeding a family or cooking for one, you can update the serving settings above to reveal the required amount of ingredients.

Atkins Yorkshire Pudding Recipe

Prep Time: 5 Minutes
Style:Other
Cook Time: 35 Minutes
Phase: Phase 3
Difficulty: Moderate

* Any adjustments made to the serving values will only update the ingredients of that recipe and not change the directions.
9.9g Protein, 12g Fat, 0.7g Fiber, 161.7kcalCalories, 3.4g Net Carbs.

INGREDIENTS
- 1/2 cup whole Grain Soy Flour
- 2 ounces vital wheat gluten
- 3 large eggs (whole)
- 1 cup whole milk
- 1 teaspoon salt
- 1/3 cup Canola Vegetable Oil
- 1 teaspoon baking powder (straight Phosphate, double acting)

DIRECTIONS
Torkshire Pudding is traditionally made with pan drippings from cooking meat. In this recipe oil is listed instead. Feel free to use pan drippings for a more flavorful pudding.

1. Preheat oven to 450° F.
2. Whisk together soy flour, gluten, eggs, milk and salt.
3. Pour drippings or oil into an 8-inch square baking dish, and place on center rack in oven for 5 minutes, until drippings or oil is smoking hot. Then add batter and bake 15 minutes.
4. Lower temperature to 350° F and bake for 15 to 20 minutes more, until lightly browned. Serve piping hot.

COOKING TIP: Having a party? When planning your low carb spread, think about which dishes you can make in advance and which need fresh ingredients that day.

Bagna Cauda Recipe

Prep Time: 5 Minutes
Style:Italian
Cook Time: 5 Minutes
Phase: Phase 1
Difficulty: Easy

* Any adjustments made to the serving values will only update the ingredients of that recipe and not change the directions.
1.3g Protein, 19.6g Fat, 0g Fiber, 180.2kcalCalories, 0.3gNet Carbs.

INGREDIENTS
• 1/2 cup extra virgin olive oil
• 1/4 cup unsalted butter stick
• 3 teaspoons garlic
• 8 each anchovy (Drained Solids In Oil, Canned)

DIRECTIONS

1. In a small saucepan, heat olive oil and butter over medium heat.

2. Add garlic and anchovies. Cook gently for 5 minutes, until garlic is fragrant (but not brown).

3. Add pepper to taste. Transfer to a hot pot or heated dish and serve with vegetables.

COOKING TIP: If you're serving as an appetizer, plate your dip with two or three different low carb snacks!

Baked Black Bass and Clams in Foil

Prep Time: 20 Minutes
Style:Asian
Cook Time: 10 Minutes
Phase: Phase 1
Difficulty: Moderate

* Any adjustments made to the serving values will only update the ingredients of that recipe and not change the directions.
39.3g Protein, 28.6g Fat, 0.6g Fiber, 435.2kcalCalories, 3.5g Net Carbs.

INGREDIENTS

- 1/2 cup extra virgin olive oil
- 4 tablespoons fish sauce
- 2 cloves garlic
- 2 tablespoons fresh lime juice
- 1/2 serving Crushed Red Pepper
- 1/2 cup sliced fennel bulk
- 1/2 cup chopped Celery
- 20 ounces Pacific cod (fish)
- 12 medium Clams

DIRECTIONS

The original recipe calls for black bass. Cod works wonderfully and easier to find. You could also use hake or another flakey white fish. Salmon also works well. Baking fish in foil has several advantages. It can be prepared ahead of time and there's no pan to clean or fishy odor in the kitchen. You also have total control of the temperature of the fish. This recipe also calls for kaffir lime leaves, they are available in Asian markets and some well-stocked supermarkets. Substitute with basil leaves or a little lime zest if you cannot find them. Additionally you will need 4 (6x8-inch) pieces of banana leaves or parchment paper.

1. Preheat oven to 375°F.

2. In a small bowl, mix together the olive oil, fish sauce, minced garlic, lime juice and red pepper flakes; set aside

3. Place pieces of foil on a clean, dry surface and top each with a banana leaf. Thinly slice the fennel and celery.

4. Divide the fennel and celery into four equal portions and place one portion of each on each banana leaf. Place 1 (5-ounce) bass filet, 3 clams and one-quarter of the kaffir lime leaves on the fennel and celery. Spoon the sauce over fish and vegetables.

5. Fold and crimp the edges of the foil to seal packets. Bake for 8-10 minutes, depending on the thickness of the fish.

6. Place each packet on a plate and serve. Be certain the clams are open before serving.

COOKING TIP: Whether you're feeding a family or cooking for one, you can update the serving settings above to reveal the required amount of ingredients.

Lemon Mousse Parfait with Lime Crema and Toasted Walnuts Recipe

Prep Time: 15 Minutes
Style:French
Cook Time: 20 Minutes
Phase: Phase 2
Difficulty: Difficult

* Any adjustments made to the serving values will only update the ingredients of that recipe and not change the directions.

9g Protein, 34.2g Fat, 1.5g Fiber, 362.3kcalCalories, 6.9g Net Carbs.

INGREDIENTS

- 1/4 cup chopped English Walnuts

- 9 tablespoons Fresh Lemon Juice

- 3 large eggs (whole)

- 3 large egg yolks

- 6 packets Stevia

- 2 tablespoons unsalted butter stick

- 3/4 cup Heavy Cream

• 5 tablespoons fresh lime juice

DIRECTIONS

This delicious dessert layers lemon curd, lime cream, and walnut for contrasts in color and texture. Use a zester, the fine side of a box grater or a micro plane to zest the lemons and limes. This recipe has been adjusted to the amount of zest and juice you will need. If you buy whole fruit then it will be 3 lemons and limes.

1. Preheat oven to 400° F. Place the walnuts on baking sheet and cook until brown, about 8 minutes, being careful not to burn.

2. Bring a large pot of water or a double boiler to a boil.

3. Zest the lemons and then juice them. Place zest and juice in a medium bowl or the top of a double boiler. Add the whole eggs and yolks. Place the bowl over the boiling water and turn heat down to low. With a hand mixer, whisk the eggs, yolks and lemon juice until mixture is creamy and doubles in volume. Remove from heat. Add

the butter and 4 packets sugar substitute to the bowl and allow the mixture to cool.

4. Place the cream in a mixing bowl. Zest and then juice the limes, as above. Add to the cream. Whisk the lime and cream mixture until soft peaks form. Add 2 packets of stevia.

5. In 4 parfait or martini glasses, layer first one-half of the lime crema, then one-third of the walnuts, followed by all the lemon curd. Next add another layer of walnuts and top them with the remaining lime crema.

COOKING TIP: We love the idea of customizing this recipe to make it your own! If you add any ingredients, just be sure to keep an eye on net carbs.

Braised Lamb Shanks with Spiced Quince Recipe

Prep Time: 35 Minutes
Style:Italian
Cook Time: 240 Minutes
Phase: Phase 3
Difficulty: Difficult

* Any adjustments made to the serving values will only update the ingredients of that recipe and not change the directions.

71.5g Protein, 52.5g Fat, 2.4g Fiber, 832kcalCalories, 11.5g Net Carbs.

INGREDIENTS

• 72 ounces lamb leg (Shank Half, Trimmed to 1/8" Fat, Choice Grade)

• 5 tablespoons canola vegetable oil

• 7 cups chicken broth, bouillon or consomme

• 2 cups sliced onions

• 10 cloves garlic

• 2 servings diced plum tomatoes

- 1/3 ounce thyme

- 1 1/4 each Bay Leaf

- 2 fruit without refuses Quinces

- 1/2 teaspoon Cinnamon

- 1/2 teaspoon whole black peppercorns

- 3 tablespoons peppermint (Mint)

DIRECTIONS

When I was growing up, my family rarely ate beef, but lamb was usually on the table, which may be why I tend to cook with it nowadays. The shank is one of my favorite cuts and is quite inexpensive. Although it takes a long time to cook, it has a delectably rich, buttery flavor and usually falls off the bone. Caramelizing the shanks before putting them in the oven further enhances the flavor of this dish. Lamb pairs well with fruit, and I usually braise in the fall and early winter when quince are in season. Looking like a cross between a pear and an apple, quince becomes sweet after cooking. Although the amount of meat may seem large, at least half of each shank is bone.

Note: You will need a 3-inch piece of cinnamon (or the 1/2 tsp ground cinnamon), 1 whole allspice berry and 2 whole cloves to make the quince sauce.

1. Preheat the oven to 325°F.

2. Season the lamb shanks with salt and pepper. Heat 3 tablespoons of canola oil in a large saute pan or skillet on high, and then add shanks. Sear for about 3-4 minutes on each side, or until golden-brown on all sides. Remove to a large braising pan.

3. Bring 1 cup of chicken broth to a boil, add to the saute pan and with the heat on low, deglaze the pan by scraping the remaining pieces of meat stuck to it with a whisk or spatula. Transfer to the braising pan with the shanks.

4. In a medium sauté pan, heat the remaining 2 tablespoons of canola oil and "sweat" the onions and garlic over medium-low heat, stirring occasionally, for about 12-14 minutes. The onions should be soft and translucent.

5. Add the tomato and 1 cup of chicken broth, bring to a simmer and then transfer

the mixture to the braising pan with the shanks.

6. Pour the remaining 4 cups of broth into the braising pan. Add the bay leaves and thyme. Cover with parchment paper or aluminum foil and a lid and place in the oven.

7. After the lamb has been cooking for about 3 hours, place the quince, 1 cup of chicken broth, cinnamon stick, peppercorns, allspice and cloves in a small sauce pot. Bring to a boil and then reduce heat and simmer for 45 minutes, or until tender. Remove the quince and keep warm. Discard the liquid and seasonings.

8. After about 4 hours of cooking, when the meat is tender and almost falling off the bone, remove the shanks from the oven and let them cool until they can be handled. (They should still be warm.) Remove the shanks from the pan, leaving the vegetables in the pan juices. Cover the shanks to keep them warm .

9. Place the braising pan on the top of the range and with two burners on medium-high, reduce the sauce by whisking it until it

is thick enough to coat a spoon for 45 minutes.

10. To serve, place one-sixth of the quince on the side of each plate with a shank next to it and lap the sauce over it. Top with mint.

COOKING TIP: Whether you're feeding a family or cooking for one, you can update the serving settings above to reveal the required amount of ingredients.

LOW CARB DESSERT RECIPES

Lemon Mousse Parfait with Lime Crema and Toasted Walnuts Recipe

Prep Time: 15 Minutes
Style:French
Cook Time: 20 Minutes
Phase: Phase 2
Difficulty: Difficult

* Any adjustments made to the serving values will only update the ingredients of that recipe and not change the directions.

9g Protein, 34.2g Fat, 1.5g Fiber, 362.3kcalCalories, 6.9g Net Carbs.

INGREDIENTS

- 1/4 cup chopped English Walnuts
- 9 tablespoons Fresh Lemon Juice
- 3 large eggs (whole)
- 3 large egg yolks
- 6 packets Stevia
- 2 tablespoons unsalted butter stick
- 3/4 cup Heavy Cream
- 5 tablespoons fresh lime juice

DIRECTIONS

This delicious dessert layers lemon curd, lime cream, and walnut for contrasts in color and texture. Use a zester, the fine side of a box grater or a micro plane to zest the lemons and limes. This recipe has been adjusted to the amount of zest and juice you will need. If you buy whole fruit then it will be 3 lemons and limes.

1. Preheat oven to 400° F. Place the walnuts on baking sheet and cook until brown, about 8 minutes, being careful not to burn.

2. Bring a large pot of water or a double boiler to a boil.

3. Zest the lemons and then juice them. Place zest and juice in a medium bowl or the top of a double boiler. Add the whole eggs and yolks. Place the bowl over the boiling water and turn heat down to low. With a hand mixer, whisk the eggs, yolks and lemon juice until mixture is creamy and doubles in volume. Remove from heat. Add the butter and 4 packets sugar substitute to the bowl and allow the mixture to cool.

4. Place the cream in a mixing bowl. Zest and then juice the limes, as above. Add to the cream. Whisk the lime and cream mixture until soft peaks form. Add 2 packets of stevia.

5. In 4 parfait or martini glasses, layer first one-half of the lime cream, then one-third of the walnuts, followed by all the lemon curd. Next add another layer of walnuts and top them with the remaining lime crema.

COOKING TIP: We love the idea of customizing this recipe to make it your own! If you add any ingredients, just be sure to keep an eye on net carbs.

Keto Almond Butter Protein Truffles

Prep Time: 55 Minutes
Style:American
Cook Time: 5 Minutes
Phase: Phase 2
Difficulty: Easy

* Any adjustments made to the serving values will only update the ingredients of that recipe and not change the directions.

3.3g Protein, 6.9g Fat, 2.3g Fiber, 82.1kcalCalories, 1.8g Net Carbs.

INGREDIENTS

• 6 tablespoons almond butter

• 6 tablespoon(s) coconut cream, canned unsweetened

• 1 scoop (1 scoop= 30 g) quest chocolate milkshake protein powder

- 3/4 teaspoon glucomannan, pure powder (1 tsp= 4 g)

- 1 dash salt

- 6 tablespoons chocolate chips, sugar free

- 1 teaspoon(s) coconut oil

DIRECTIONS

1. In a medium mixing bowl, mix the almond butter, coconut cream, and salt together until well combined. If both the almond butter and coconut cream are solid or cold, you may need to warm them either in the microwave (in a microwaves safe container) or over a pot of steaming water (in a heat proof bowl) to be able to completely incorporate.

2. Add the protein powder, glucomannan (or other finely ground fiber source), and mix until all the powder is worked in, and a smooth texture develops. The mixture will be slightly oily.

3. Line a baking sheet with parchment paper. Make 14 tablespoon mounds of the almond butter mixture on the parchment

paper lined baking sheet and put into the freezer to cool for 10 minutes, or until chilled enough to form into a ball. Form into balls and freeze until well set, another 20 minutes.

4. While the balls are cooling, use a double boiler (or in a medium heat proof bowl over a small saucepan with about 1-inch simmering water) to melt the chocolate chips and coconut oil together, stirring until fully melted and uniform texture. Keep warm until the balls are well cooled.

5. Remove the balls from the freezer and, one at a time, roll in the melted chocolate to coat. Place each coated truffle back on the parchment paper and refrigerate until the chocolate has hardened, about 10 minutes. Store in an airtight container in the refrigerator for up to one week. One truffle is one serving.

COOKING TIP: Try adding diced freeze dried strawberries as a variation. Adding in 1-2 freeze dried strawberry slices won't change the NC of this naturally keto and low carb recipe enough to worry about so just enjoy!

Apricot-Apple Cloud Recipe

Prep Time: 65 Minutes
Style:American
Cook Time: 0 Minutes
Phase: Phase 3
Difficulty: Easy

* Any adjustments made to the serving
values will only update the ingredients of
that recipe and not change the directions.
1.4g Protein, 22.2g Fat, 1.4g Fiber,
241.7kcalCalories, 9.8g Net Carbs.

INGREDIENTS
• 1 1/2 cups heavy cream
• 2 tablespoons sucralose based sweetener
(Sugar Substitute)
• 16 ounces Baby Food Applesauce and
Apricots

DIRECTIONS

This no-cook dessert uses a surprise ingredient: baby food. Be sure to use a product without added sugar and to allow at least an hour to chill the dessert.

1. With an electric mixer on medium, beat cream and sugar substitute until medium-firm peaks form.
2. Gently fold in baby food (you will need 16 oz or four 4 oz jars).
3. Divide among 6 dessert glasses and chill at least 1 hour before serving.

COOKING TIP: We love the idea of customizing this recipe to make it your own! If you add any ingredients, just be sure to keep an eye on net carbs.

Atkins Cinnamon Pie Crust Recipe

Prep Time: 10 Minutes
Style:American
Cook Time: 0 Minutes
Phase: Phase 3
Difficulty: Easy

* Any adjustments made to the serving values will only update the ingredients of that recipe and not change the directions.
9g Protein, 13.5g Fat, 1.6g Fiber, 168.4kcalCalories, 2.4g Net Carbs

INGREDIENTS
- 1/4 teaspoon salt
- 1 teaspoon sucralose based sweetener (sugar substitute)
- 1 teaspoon cinnamon
- 1/2 cup unsalted butter stick
- 2 tablespoons tap water
- 3 3/4 servings Atkins Flour Mix

DIRECTIONS
Use the Atkins recipe to make Atkins Flour Mix. You will need 1 1/4 cups to make one pie crust.

1. Pulse the baking mix, salt, sugar substitute, and cinnamon in a food processor to incorporate; add butter and pulse until mixture resembles a coarse meal, about 30 seconds. Pulse in water until dough just comes together, about 30 seconds (add up to 1 more tablespoon if necessary).
2. Transfer dough to a sheet of plastic wrap; form into a disk about 6 inches in diameter.

Wrap tightly in plastic; refrigerate until firm, about 30 minutes.
3. Roll and bake as directed in pie recipe. Makes 1 pie crust.

Find this recipe and more in the New Atkins For a New You Cookbook!

COOKING TIP: We love the idea of customizing this recipe to make it your own! If you add any ingredients, just be sure to keep an eye on net carbs.

Berries with Chocolate Ganache Recipe

Prep Time: 10 Minutes
Style:French
Cook Time: 5 Minutes
Phase: Phase 2
Difficulty: Easy

* Any adjustments made to the serving values will only update the ingredients of that recipe and not change the directions.
4g Protein, 17.6g Fat, 8.1g Fiber, 286.3kcalCalories, 9.5g Net Carbs.

INGREDIENTS
- 8 ounces strawberries
- 2 cups red raspberries
- 2 cups fresh blueberries
- 8 ounces sugar free chocolate chips
- 1/3 cup heavy cream
- 1/2 teaspoon vanilla extract

DIRECTIONS
1. Combine fruit and place into 6 dessert bowls.
2. In a small saucepan over low heat, heat chocolate and cream until just melted (this can be done in a microwave for 30 seconds at a time. Be careful not to overheat and burn the chocolate). Add vanilla and stir until smooth.
3. Cool slightly and drizzle sauce over fruit just before serving.

COOKING TIP: We love the idea of customizing this recipe to make it your own! If you add any ingredients, just be sure to keep an eye on net carbs.

Blackberry-Orange Sorbet Recipe

Prep Time: 240 Minutes
Style:American
Cook Time: 20 Minutes
Phase: Phase 3
Difficulty: Easy

* Any adjustments made to the serving values will only update the ingredients of that recipe and not change the directions.
3.6g Protein, 1.6g Fat, 4.3g Fiber, 75.9kcalCalories, 8.5g Net Carbs.

INGREDIENTS
• 2 1/4 cups blackberries
• 1 teaspoon orange zest
• 1 cup buttermilk (Reduced Fat, Cultured)
• 1/3 cup sucralose based sweetener (Sugar Substitute)

DIRECTIONS
1. In a medium saucepan, bring blackberries, sugar substitute, 2 tablespoons water, and orange zest to a boil. Reduce heat and simmer, covered, for 15 minutes, stirring

occasionally, until berries break down. Cool quickly by placing in a bowl sitting in another larger bowl filled with an ice water bath.

2. Place cooled berry mixture in a food processor. Process until smooth. Press through a fine strainer into a bowl. Stir in buttermilk. Chill in refrigerator 1 hour or until cold.

3. Pour into an ice-cream maker and run according to manufacturer's directions. Transfer to a bowl and freeze 2 to 3 hours before serving. 1 serving is about 1/2 cup.

COOKING TIP: We love the idea of customizing this recipe to make it your own! If you add any ingredients, just be sure to keep an eye on net carbs.

Blueberry and Almond Protein Mousse Recipe

Prep Time: 15 Minutes
Style: American
Cook Time: 0 Minutes
Phase: Phase 2
Difficulty: Easy

* Any adjustments made to the serving values will only update the ingredients of that recipe and not change the directions.
4.9g Protein, 20.4g Fat, 1.9g Fiber, 222.7kcalCalories, 5.1g Net Carbs

INGREDIENTS
• 4 tablespoons cream cheese, original
• 28 grams Atkins vanilla protein powder
• 1 cup, fluid (yields 2 cups whipped) heavy whipping cream
• 1/3 teaspoon almond extract
• 1 cup blueberries, fresh
• 1/4 cup sliced almonds

DIRECTIONS

1. With an electric mixer blend together the softened cream cheese and protein powder until smooth. Set aside.

2. In a separate bowl whip the heavy cream with the almond extract until doubled in volume.

3. Gently add 1/3 of the whipped cream to the cream cheese mixture blending by hand until smooth. Add another 3rd of the whipped cream folding it into the mixture until well blended. Add the final 3rd of the whipped cream, folding until fully incorporated. Divide into 6 serving bowls, cover with plastic wrap and refrigerate until ready to serve.

4. To toast the almonds, place them on a sheet pan and toast for 3-5 minutes at 350°F. Sprinkle each bowl with blueberries and sliced almonds before serving.

COOKING TIP: We love the idea of customizing this recipe to make it your own! If you add any ingredients, just be sure to keep an eye on net carbs.

Cafe Caramel Panna Cotta

Prep Time: 5 Minutes
Style:American
Cook Time: 10 Minutes
Phase: Phase 2
Difficulty: Easy

* Any adjustments made to the serving values will only update the ingredients of that recipe and not change the directions.
4.7g Protein, 23.5g Fat, 0.2g Fiber, 237.8kcalCalories, 2.1g Net Carbs.

INGREDIENTS
- 1 envelope gelatin, unsweetened
- 2 tablespoons tap water
- 1 1/2 cups Heavy Cream, liquid
- 1 each Atkins café caramel shake
- 3 tablespoons confectioners (powdered) erythritol
- 5 drops liquid stevia drops
- 1 teaspoon vanilla extract

Ingredient note: We recommend using English Toffee flavored liquid stevia drops for this recipe.

DIRECTIONS

1. In a cup, sprinkle the gelatin onto the water and set aside.

2. In a small saucepan, whisk together the cream, shake, sweeteners and vanilla. Warm over medium heat, stirring occasionally, until just starting to simmer, about 10 minutes.

3. Remove from heat, and whisk in the gelatin until dissolved. Fill 6 ramekins with ½ cup of the liquid, cover with plastic wrap, and refrigerate for at least 3 hours or until the gelatin is set.

OPTIONAL: serve with a dollop of whipped cream (1 tablespoon adds .021 net carbs), or a teaspoon of sugar free caramel syrup (does not add net carbs).

VARIATIONS: We developed this recipe using the Café Caramel shake, but you could substitute any other shake for a wealth of flavor options.

LOW CARB BEVERAGE RECIPES

Almond-Pineapple Smoothie Recipe

Prep Time: 5 Minutes
Style:American
Cook Time: Minutes
Phase: Phase 3
Difficulty: Easy

* Any adjustments made to the serving values will only update the ingredients of that recipe and not change the directions.
10.7g Protein, 17.3g Fat, 3.9g Fiber, 275.7kcalCalories, 16.1g Net Carbs.

INGREDIENTS
• 1/2 cup (8 fluid ounces) plain yogurt (whole milk)
• 2 1/2 ounces pineapple
• 20 each wholes blanched & slivered almonds
• 1/2 cup pure almond milk - unsweetened original

DIRECTIONS

Feel free to substitute other fruits or nuts for the pineapple and/or almonds (about 20 whole almonds, 3 Tbsp slivered). Be sure to use fresh pineapple in this smoothie. Canned pineapple is swimming in sugar.

Combine the yogurt, pineapple, almonds and almond milk in a blender and purée until smooth and creamy.

COOKING TIP: Whether you're feeding a family or cooking for one, you can update the serving settings above to reveal the required amount of ingredients.

Atkins Chocolate Slushies Recipe

Prep Time: 5 Minutes
Style:American
Cook Time: 10 Minutes
Phase: Phase 1
Difficulty: Easy

* Any adjustments made to the serving values will only update the ingredients of that recipe and not change the directions.
2.8g Protein, 22.4g Fat, 1.9g Fiber, 229.5kcalCalories, 6.4g Net Carbs.

INGREDIENTS
• 1 cup Heavy Cream
• 1/2 cup tap water
• 2 tablespoons cocoa powder (unsweetened)
• 1/2 cup Sugar Free Chocolate Syrup
• 1 teaspoon vanilla extract

DIRECTIONS
1. In a medium saucepan combine cream, water, cocoa powder and 1/2 cup unsweetened chocolate syrup.
2. Bring to a boil over medium heat. Reduce heat to low; cook, stirring occasionally, 5 minutes. Remove from heat and stir in vanilla.

3. Pour mixture into two ice cube trays. Freeze 2 hours.

4. Before serving transfer cubes into a food processor. Pulse until mixture is finely chopped and slushy.

COOKING TIP: Why not have friends over to enjoy this drink! Update the serving settings above to reveal the required amount of ingredients you'll need.

Almond Raspberry Smoothie Recipe

Prep Time: 5 Minutes
Style:American
Cook Time: Minutes
Phase: Phase 2
Difficulty: Easy

* Any adjustments made to the serving values will only update the ingredients of that recipe and not change the directions.
18.2g Protein, 13.7g Fat, 6.9g Fiber, 259.4kcalCalories, 10.3g Net Carbs.

INGREDIENTS
- 4 ounces Greek Yogurt - Plain (Container)
- 1/2 cup Red Raspberries
- 20 each wholes Blanched & Slivered almonds
- 1/2 cup pure almond milk - unsweetened original

DIRECTIONS
Feel free to come up with your own combination of other berries and nuts for this protein-packed smoothie. If you use frozen raspberries, make sure they contain no added sugar.

Combine the yogurt, raspberries, almonds and almond milk in a blender and purée until smooth and creamy.

COOKING TIP: Whether you're feeding a family or cooking for one, you can update the serving settings above to reveal the required amount of ingredients.

Avocado Gazpacho Smoothie Recipe

Prep Time: 5 Minutes
Style:Mexican
Cook Time: 0 Minutes
Phase: Phase 1
Difficulty: Easy

* Any adjustments made to the serving values will only update the ingredients of that recipe and not change the directions.
9.1g Protein, 38.2g Fat, 11.9g Fiber, 419.5kcalCalories, 4.7g Net Carbs.

 INGREDIENTS
• 1 fruit without skin and seed California Avocado
• 1 ounce goat cheese (Soft)
• 1 tablespoon heavy cream
• 2 teaspoons fresh lime juice
• 1/8 teaspoon salt
• 1 cup Tap water
• 2 teaspoons chopped chives

DIRECTIONS

1. Place cut-up avocado in a blender. Add remaining ingredients, and blend until smooth. If needed, add additional water, 1 tablespoon at a time, to reach desired consistency.

2. Pour into a tall glass, and garnish with chives and a reserved slice of avocado, if desired. Serve immediately.

COOKING TIP: Whether you're feeding a family or cooking for one, you can update the serving settings above to reveal the required amount of ingredients.

Hazelnut Hot Chocolate Recipe

Prep Time: 5 Minutes
Style:American
Cook Time: 2 Minutes
Phase: Phase 1
Difficulty: Easy

* Any adjustments made to the serving values will only update the ingredients of that recipe and not change the directions.
17.9g Protein, 20.9g Fat, 5.9g Fiber, 286.1kcalCalories, 3.5g Net Carbs.

INGREDIENTS
• 14 nuts Hazelnuts
• 1/4 teaspoon vanilla extract
• 1 each Atkins Dark Chocolate Royale Shake

DIRECTIONS

1. Place chopped hazelnuts, vanilla (can substitute hazelnut extract for more hazelnut flavor) and 1/3 of the shake into a blender and blend on high until creamy and all the hazelnuts have been broken down; about 30 seconds. Add the remaining shake and blend until smooth.

2. Pour into a sauce pan and heat gently over medium heat while stirring until hot but not boiling. Pour into a mug and enjoy with a sprinkle of ground cinnamon.

NOTE: This may also be heated in a microwave but do so at 30 second intervals as it will foam with heating and may overflow your cup.

COOKING TIP: We love the idea of customizing this recipe to make it your own! If you add any ingredients, just be sure to keep an eye on net carbs.

Gin Fizz Recipe

Prep Time: 0 Minutes
Style:American
Cook Time: 0 Minutes
Phase: Phase 2
Difficulty: Easy

* Any adjustments made to the serving values will only update the ingredients of that recipe and not change the directions.
4.6g Protein, 16.6g Fat, 0.1g Fiber, 252.2kcalCalories, 3.3g Net Carbs.

INGREDIENTS
• 1 fluid ounce (no ice) Gin
• 1 wedge lime juice
• 1 wedge Lemon juice
• 1/2 teaspoon orange zest
• 1 packet no calorie sweetener packets
• 1 large white egg
• 3 tablespoons Heavy Cream
• 1/4 serving Original Seltzer Water (Can)

DIRECTIONS

For Cocktail: Shake all except seltzer in a cocktail mixer with ice. Strain into a cocktail glass, top off with seltzer and garnish with ground cinnamon and freshly grated nutmeg. Note that you will need about 1 tsp each of the lemon and lime juice.

It is best to use pasteurized eggs for this recipe. They can be hard to find except during the holiday months.

To pasteurze: place room temperature large eggs in a small saucepan covered with cold water. (Be sure they are at room temperature otherwise they will not get warm enough to pasteurize through to the yolk.) Place pan on the stove and cook over medium heat. Bring water to 140°F (but not higher than 145°F). It is best to use a thermometer but if you don't have a thermometer, 150° F is right about the time bubbles begin forming on the bottom of the pan. Allow the eggs to stay at that temperature for 3 minutes then quickly remove from the pan and cool under coldwater. Refrigerate until ready to use.

COOKING TIP: Why not have friends over to enjoy this drink? Update the serving settings above to reveal the required amount of ingredients you'll need.

Frozen Mocha Slushie Recipe

Prep Time: 5 Minutes
Style:American
Cook Time: 2 Minutes
Phase: Phase 1
Difficulty: Easy

* Any adjustments made to the serving values will only update the ingredients of that recipe and not change the directions.
2.3g Protein, 22.8g Fat, 1.8g Fiber, 225.7kcalCalories, 4.9g Net Carbs.

INGREDIENTS
• 4 fluid ounces decaffeinated coffee
• 3 tablespoons sugar-free chocolate syrup, Hershey's
• 2 tablespoons cocoa powder (Unsweetened)
• 2 teaspoons No Calorie Sweetener
• 1/2 cup Heavy Cream

DIRECTIONS

This recipe is a too high in NC for phase 1 but if you make only half a serving as a dessert or treat it is acceptable.

1. In a small saucepan over medium heat, stir together the coffee, chocolate syrup and cocoa powder. Stir until cocoa has dissolved, about 2 minutes. Cool slightly.

2. Transfer to a blender. Add sugar substitute and cream; blend until combined. Add 12 to 14 ice cubes in batches; blending until frothy.

COOKING TIP: Why not have friends over to enjoy this drink? Update the serving settings above to reveal the required amount of ingredients you'll need.

Cinnamon Spiced Coconut-Vanilla Protein Shake Recipe

Prep Time: 5 Minutes
Style:American
Cook Time: 0 Minutes
Phase: Phase 1
Difficulty: Easy

* Any adjustments made to the serving values will only update the ingredients of that recipe and not change the directions.
25g Protein, 4.5g Fat, 1.6g Fiber, 164.1kcalCalories, 2.6g Net Carbs.

INGREDIENTS
- 3 ice cubes (3/4 fluid ounce) water
- 1 cup Coconut milk unsweetened
- 1 ounce or scoop vanilla whey protein
- 1/2 teaspoon cinnamon
- 1/2 teaspoon vanilla extract

DIRECTIONS
1. Combine all ingredients in a blender and blend until smooth. If your protein powder does not have stevia or another granulated sugar substitute consider adding up to 1 teaspoon (add .5g NC) of sucralose (add .5g NC to the total grams of NC) or xylitol (no

additional g NC need to be added for xylitol or additional stevia).

COOKING TIP: Whether you're feeding a family or cooking for one, you can update the serving settings above to reveal the required amount of ingredients.

Extra-Creamy Strawberry Shake Recipe

Prep Time: 5 Minutes
Style:American
Cook Time: 0 Minutes
Phase: Phase 2
Difficulty: Easy

* Any adjustments made to the serving values will only update the ingredients of that recipe and not change the directions.
26.5g Protein, 22.1g Fat, 0.7g Fiber, 336.2kcalCalories, 5.9g Net Carbs.

INGREDIENTS
- 6 medium (1-1/4" diameter) Strawberries
- 2 scoops strawberry whey protein
- 1/2 cup heavy cream
- 1 teaspoon vanilla extract
- 2 cups tap water
- 2 individual packets sucralose based sweetener (sugar substitute)

DIRECTIONS
1. Place strawberries, protein powder, cream, vanilla, water, and sugar substitute in a blender and blend at high speed until very smooth.

COOKING TIP: Whether you're feeding a family or cooking for one, you can update the serving settings above to reveal the required amount of ingredients.

RENAL DIET COOKBOOK FOR BEGINNERS #2021:

Comprehensive Guide With One Year of Low Potassium and Low Sodium Recipes to Manage Kidney Disease (Ckd), Start Off Your Day and Avoid Dialysis

AUTHOR

CHARLOTTE CONLAN

TABLE OF CONTENTS

WHAT IS KIDNEY DISEASE?

Kidney disease is very common. However, less than 1 in 10 of the people with kidney disease develop failure of the kidneys requiring dialysis or a kidney transplant.

Even though they may never develop completly kidney problems, people with kidney disease will benefit from tests to see if they are likely to develop problems in the future. If the blood pressure is high, it should be treated to protect the kidneys against further damage and to reduce the risk of stroke or heart attack.

Kidney disease is a term used by doctors to include any abnormality of the kidneys, even if there is only very slight damage. It is often called 'chronic' kidney disease. Chronic is a medical term that means a condition that does not get completly better in a few days. A problem with the kidneys, such as an uncomplicated urine infection, that gets better and leaves no damage, is not chronic kidney disease.

What is kidney failure?

Kidney failure is a medical term that can be confusing, because it refers to reduced kidney function, usually less than 30% of normal (or estimated kidney function of less than 30). Some people with kidney failure feel perfectly well, and in some cases the kidneys can continue to work for some years without deteriorating to a serious level.

CHRONIC KIDNEY DISEASE (CKD)

Kidney disease is a term used by doctors to include any abnormality of the kidneys, even if there is only very slight damage. 'Chronic' means a condition that does not get completly better. Some people think that 'chronic' means severe. This is not the case, and often CKD is only a very slight abnormality in the kidneys.

HOW COMMON IS CKD?

Research suggests that 1 in 10 of the population may have CKD, but it is less common in young adults, infact it is present in 1 in 50 people. In those aged over 75 years old, CKD is present in 1 out of 2 people. However, many of the elderly people with CKD may not have 'diseased' kidneys, but have normal aging of their kidneys. Although severe kidney failure will not occur with normal ageing of the kidneys, there is an increased chance of high blood pressure and heart disease or stroke, so medical checks will be helpful.

HOW DO YOU KNOW IF YOU HAVE CKD?

In most cases CKD does not cause any symptoms, and is detected because tests are abnormal. These may be urine tests for blood or protein; an X-ray or scan of the kidneys; or a blood test to measure kidney function.

WHAT CAUSES CKD?

There are many causes of CKD, and two of the commonest causes are high blood pressure and aging of the kidneys. Very few of the causes of CKD are completely curable, so it is often not necessary to do extensive tests to find a cause, so long as blood tests show the kidney function is stable. If someone has markedly reduced kidney function, declining kidney function, or associated problems such as kidney pain, a scan of the kidneys will be performed. Some people will also have tests such as a cystoscopy (flexible tube to look inside the bladder), or a kidney biopsy (a small piece of kidney is removed with a needle and looked at under the microscope).

Kidney disease is most often caused by poorly controlled diabetes or high blood pressure. Physical injurys and drug toxicity can also damage your kidneys.

Uncontrolled diabetes is the leading cause of kidney failure. Diabetes develops when blood glucose (blood sugar) levels are too high in the body. When our bodies digest protein from the food we eat, the process of digestion creates waste products. In the kidneys, millions of tiny blood vessels, called capillaries, act as filters. As blood flows through the capillaries, the waste products are filtered out into our urine. Substances such as protein and red blood cells are too big to pass through the capillaries and stay in the blood.

Diabetes damages this process. High levels of sugar in the blood make the kidneys filter too much blood. All the extra work wears down the filters, and after many years the filters start to leak. The good protein our bodies need is then filtered out and lost through the urine. Eventually, the kidneys cannot remove the extra waste from the blood. This ultimately leads to kidney damage or failure. This damage can happen over many years without any signs or symptoms. That is why it is so important for people with diabetes to manage their blood-sugar levels and get tested for kidney disease periodically.

SYMPTOMS

Kidney failure is a progressive disease; it does not happen overnight. Some people in the early stages of kidney disease don't show any symptoms. Symptoms usually appear in the later stages of kidney disease. Some people may not even show any symptoms of kidney disease until their kidneys fail (end stage).

When the kidneys are damaged, wastes and toxins can build up in your body. Once the buildup starts to occur, you may feel sick and experience some of the following symptoms:

Nausea

Poor appetite, weakness, trouble sleeping, tiredness

Itching Weight loss

Muscle cramps (especially in the legs) , swelling of your feet and ankles anemia (low red blood cell count)

WHAT ARE THE STAGES OF CKD?

CKD is divided into 5 stages:

- CKD stage 1 is eGFR greater than 90 mls/min, which is normal but there are some signs of kidney damage on other tests (if all the other kidney tests are normal, there is no CKD).
- CKD stage 2 is eGFR 60-90. This is mildly decreased with some sign of kidney damage (if all the kidney tests are normal, there is no CKD).
- CKD stage 3a is eGFR 45-59 ml/min, a mild to moderate reduction in kidney function
- CKD stage 3b is eGFR 30-44 ml/min, a moderate to severe reduction in kidney function

- CKD stage 4 is eGFR 15-29 ml/min, a severe reduction in kidney function
- CKD stage 5 is e GFR less than 15 ml/min, established kidney failure, when dialysis or a kidney transplant may be needed.

THE TREATMENT FOR CKD?

There are some things that everyone with CKD should try to do. These are:-

- Lose weight (if overweight), and take regular exercise
- Stop smoking
- Reduce the amount of salt in the diet in order to help control the blood pressure.
- Eat a healthy balanced diet
- Drink about 2 litres of fluid a day (2 litres is about 10 cups or 6 mugs). There is no benefit in drinking large amounts of fluid, except in people who get lots of urine infections, or in a few other special cases
- Consider buying an automatic blood pressure monitor to check the blood pressure at home

- Have an annual 'flu jab (influenza vaccination), and have the pneumonia (pneumococcal) vaccine once (talk to your GP about this)
- Avoid taking medications which can harm the kidney and increase blood pressure, such as some anti-inflammatory medications.

The blood pressure should be treated carefully. If it is above 140/85, tablets are usually needed, and the aim is to get the blood pressure down to 140/90 or lower if you have proteinuria or have diabetes. The cholesterol level should be checked, and some people will be advised to take a daily aspirin tablet. A blood test to check eGFR should be performed once a year. If the urine tests show a lot of protein in the urine, or the kidney function is declining over time, the case will be discussed with a kidney specialist, or a referral may be made to a kidney specialist.

TREATMENT FOR CKD STAGE 3A AND 3B

In these stages the desease is treats as in CKD stages 1 and 2, but with more careful monitoring for declining kidney function.

TREATMENT FOR CKD STAGES 4 AND 5

In these stages the desease is treats as for CKD stages 1-3. Additionally, any medications should be reviewed, as the dose may need to be altered and some drugs may need to be avoided as they could damage the kidneys further. This should include prescribed drugs and any drugs bought at the chemist and complementary therapies. In CKD stages 4 and 5 it is usually necessary to get advice from a kidney specialist, especially in stage 5 because kidney failure may become life threatening.

THE BENEFITS OF A RENAL DIET

It is important to keep kidneys in good working order, or working at an optimum level, because they serve an important function. People might think the kidneys do nothing more than help eliminate urine and other waste such as ammonia and toxins from the body, but their work includes helping the body to create red blood cells and holding blood pressure steady. To do all this work, these organs use about one-fifth of the body's blood supply.

The benefits, however, are often considered by the medical community to outweigh the risks. Failure to follow such a diet, if prescribed by a doctor, could result in the progression or development of renal failure. Patients are often advised to consult a special dietitian, known as a renal dietitian, to help them better understand what their bodies need and craft an eating plan they can live with. A renal dietitian also can guide patients to the correct supplements their bodies need.

The levels of protein, phosphorus and potassium in the body are surely concern to people with kidney problems. If the kidneys aren't working as they should, levels of these substances can become unbalanced and cause serious illness. The renal diet helps a patient to limit protein to the correct amount, and preserve bone strength by ensuring there is not too much phosphorous present. Excess potassium can affect a patient's heartbeat.

The level of sodium in the body is also surely concern for a person with kidney problems, and a renal diet can help regulate the sodium level. Patients will not excrete adequate amounts of fluid from the body if their diets do not pay specific attention to sodium and the amount of liquid they drink. Failure to comply with recommended sodium and fluid intake levels could result in the retaining of fluid and swelling of areas of the body, such as the legs, and this can cause pain. This is especially true in the later stages of kidney disease.

COMMON INGREDIENTS IN A KiDNEY FAILURE DIET FOR PRE-DIALYSIS

While there are several kidney failure diet plans available today for those with renal failure, most of them have some ingredients in common. Proteins can worsen the kidney disease to a good extent if they are eating in excess, so their intake should be minimal during stages 1 – 4 of kidney failure. Once the dialysis program has started, the protein intake should be increased.

Sodium, potassium, phosphorous and fluid intake are the other factors that should be controlled. Sodium is the most important factor to consider while choosing a kidney failure diet. Most foods contain sodium in small amounts. The assistance of a professional dietitian should be sought in order to control the intake of sodium and other needed nutrients.

FOOD TO AVOID AND FOOD TO EAT WHILE ON THE RENAL DIET

A renal diet eating plan (also called a kidney disease diet) is one that restricts sodium, potassium and phosphorus intake, since people with kidney disease/kidney issues need to monitor how much of these nutrients they consume.

Here there are some of the best foods to eat for people with kidney disease:

- **Red bell peppers:** This vegetable is low in potassium, making it ideal for the kidney diet. Red bell peppers are also a great source of vitamin C and A as well as vitamin B6. They are also a great source of lycopene, an antioxidant that protects against certain cancers.

- **Cabbage:** These vegetables are packed with phytochemicals that help break up free radicals before they can do damage. These chemicals are also known for they protective action against cancer as well as being great for cardiovascular health. Cabbage is a great source of vitamin K and C and it has an abundant amount of fiber.

- **Cauliflower:** Being rich in vitamin C and a good source of folate and fiber, cauliflower can be a great addition to any diet. This vegetable is packed with indoles, glucosinolates, and thiocyanates—elements that help the liver to neutralize toxic substances that could potentially damage cell membranes and DNA.
- **Garlic:** This aromatic food can help prevent plaque formation on your teeth, lower cholesterol, and even help reduce inflammation.
- **Onions:** Rice in flavonoids, especially quercetin, which is a powerful antioxidant that works to reduce heart disease and protects against many cancers. Onions are known for being low in potassium and a good source of chromium—a mineral that helps with carbohydrate, fat, and protein metabolism.
- **Apples:** they help to reduce cholesterol, prevent constipation, protect against heart disease, and

reduce cancer risk. Apples even contain anti-inflammatory elements that are great for reducing inflammation.

- **Cherries:** Packed with antioxidant and phytochemicals, helping protect the heart. Cherries have also been shown that they reduce inflammation when eaten daily.
- **Red grapes:** Known for containing several flavonoids to give it is characteristic red color, it helps to protect against heart disease by way of preventing oxidation and reducing the formation of blood clots.
- **Ginger:** Known for having analgesic, sedative, antipyretic, and antibacterial properties, ginger can be a great addition to any diet. It also contains vitamin B5, magnesium, and manganese. Ginger can be used to help treat joint pain and also reduces nausea
- **Coriander:** This herb has a pleasant aroma and flavor making it a wonderful addition to many food dishes. It is a good source of vitamins A, C, B2, and K. It also

packed with calcium, selenium, iron, manganese, and fiber.

FOOD TO AVOID IN A RENAL DIET

Kidney failure patients should avoid foods that are high in phosphorus or sodium. Some examples include biscuits, muffins, pancakes, waffles, oatmeal, cookies, pretzels, deli-style meat, processed cheese, canned fish, artichokes, spinach, potatoes, fresh beets, dates, oranges, frozen dinners, seasoned salts, soy sauce, and other condiments and sauces.

Here there is a list of items you should avoid on a renal diet divided by food group category.

Starches:

- 1 small biscuit or muffin
- 2 x 2-inch square of cake
- 1 (4-inch) pancake or waffle
- ½ cup of oatmeal
- ½ cup of whole-wheat cereal or bran cereal
- 1 piece of cornbread

- ¾ ounce of salted pretzel sticks or rings
- 4 sandwich cookies

Vegetables:

- Artichoke or ¼ of a whole avocado
- Brussels sprouts or okra
- Potatoes
- Spinach
- Sweet potato (Sweet potatoes have 40 mg of phosphorus or more per serving.)
- Tomatoes, regular and low-sodium tomato juice, or ¼ cup of tomato sauce
- Winter squash
- Fresh Beets

Fruit:

- 1 cup of canned or fresh apricots, or 5 dried apricots
- 1 small nectarine (2 inches across)
- 1 small orange or ½ cup of orange juice
- ¼ cup of dates
- ⅛ of a small honeydew melon
- 1 small banana

- ½ cup of prune juice or 5 dried prunes

Fats and meat:

- 1 teaspoon butter

- 2 tablespoons coconut

- 1 tablespoon powdered coffee creamer

- 1 teaspoon solid shortening

- 1 ounce of deli-style meat, such as roast beef, ham, or turkey

- 1 ounce of canned salmon or sardines

- ¼ cup of cottage cheese

- Processed cheese, such as American cheese and cheese spreads

- Smoked or cured meat, such as corned beef, bacon, ham, hot dogs, and sausage

Others:

- Frozen dinners, soups, and fast foods, such as hamburgers and pizza (see the food label for serving sizes)
- Seasoned salt, such as onion or garlic salt

- Barbecue sauce, ketchup, mustard, and chili sauce
- 2 medium green olives or 3 large black olives
- Soy sauce, steak sauce, and teriyaki sauce

OTHER FOODS TO AVOID FOR HEALTHY KIDNEYS

You should also avoid soda, processed deli meats, butter, mayonnaise, and frozen meals. These foods don't provide nutritional benefits and tend to be high in calories, sugar, and salt, which are all hazardous to the kidneys.

RENAL DIET RECIPES
BREAKFAST RECIPES

APPLE-CHAI SMOOTHIE

Serves 2/ Prep time: 5 minutes, plus 30 minutes to steep; Cook time: 5 minutes

Chai is redolent with warm spices such as ginger, cardamom, black peppercorns, fennel, cinnamon, and cloves. This tea is not only delicious but also a powerful antioxidant and may help support digestion. The taste of this smoothie is dependent on steeping the tea for at least 30 minutes.

Ingredients

1 cup unsweetened rice milk

1 chai tea bag

1 apple, peeled, cored, and chopped

2 cups ice

Directions

1. In a medium saucepan, heat the rice milk over low heat for about 5 minutes or until steaming.

2. Remove the milk from the heat and add the tea bag to steep.

3. Let the milk cool in the refrigerator with the tea bag for about 30 minutes and then remove tea bag, squeezing gently to release all the flavor.

4. Place the milk, apple, and ice in a blender and blend until smooth.

5. Pour into 2 glasses and serve.

PER SERVING Calories: 88; Fat: 1g; Carbohydrates: 19g; Phosphorus: 74mg; Potassium: 92mg; Sodium: 47mg; Protein: 1g

BLUEBERRY-PINEAPPLE SMOOTHIE

Serves 2 / Prep time: 15 minutes

The sweetness in this smoothie comes from the pineapple, so if you enjoy a more tart breakfast drink, reduce the amount you use, or use slightly underripe fruit. If you are cutting up a fresh pineapple, remove the fibrous core before adding the fruit to your blender. Pineapple is an excellent source of vitamin C and a good source of dietary fibre, vitamin B6, and copper.

Ingredients

1 cup frozen blueberries
½ cup pineapple chunks
½ cup English cucumber
½ apple
½ cup water

Directions

1. Put the blueberries, pineapple, cucumber, apple, and water in a blender and blend until thick and smooth.
2. Pour into 2 glasses and serve.

PER SERVING Calories: 87; Fat: 1g; Carbohydrates: 22g; Phosphorus: 28mg; Potassium: 192mg; Sodium: 3mg; Protein: 1g

WATERMELON-RASPBERRY SMOOTHIE

Serves 2 / Prep time: 10 minutes

The rosy pink color of this smoothie is delightful, and its breezy taste is a refreshing way to start your day. Try to keep the pale green inner rind of the watermelon when you cut it up for the smoothie, because 95 percent of its nutrition is found in that part of the melon. Watermelon is an excellent source of vitamins A and C and the antioxidants lycopene and beta-carotene.

Ingredients

½ cup boiled, cooled, and shredded red cabbage

1 cup diced watermelon

½ cup fresh raspberries

1 cup ice

Directions

1. Put the cabbage in a blender and pulse for 2 minutes or until it is finely chopped.

2. Add the watermelon and raspberries and pulse for about 1 minute or until very well combined.

3. Add the ice and blend until the smoothie is very thick and smooth.

4. Pour into 2 glasses and serve.

DIALYSIS MODIFICATION: The watermelon can be reduced by ½ cup to decrease the amount of potassium per serving by 50 mg.

PER SERVING Calories: 47; Fat: 0g; Carbohydrates: 11g; Phosphorus: 30mg; Potassium: 197mg; Sodium: 4mg; Protein: 1g

FESTIVE BERRY PARFAIT

Serves 4 / Prep time: 20 minutes, plus 1 hour to chill

Dust off your old sundae glasses, because these parfaits are spectacular when you see all the layers. Snowy cream cheese, crumbled golden cookies, and vibrant berries combine to create a breakfast for holiday weekends or even a festive dessert. The fruit layer can be anything from stewed rhubarb to peach slices or raspberries. You also can swap out the homemade meringue cookies with plain vanilla wafers.

Ingredients

1 cup vanilla rice milk, at room temperature
½ cup plain cream cheese, at room temperature
1 tablespoon granulated sugar
½ teaspoon ground cinnamon
1 cup crumbled Meringue Cookies (here)
2 cups fresh blueberries
1 cup sliced fresh strawberries

Directions

1. In a small bowl, whisk together the milk, cream cheese, sugar, and cinnamon until smooth.

2. Into 4 (6-ounce) glasses, spoon ¼ cup of crumbled cookie in the bottom of each.

3. Spoon ¼ cup of the cream cheese mixture on top of the cookies.

4. Top the cream cheese with ¼ cup of the berries.

5. Repeat in each cup with the cookies, cream cheese mixture, and berries.

6. Chill in the refrigerator for 1 hour and serve.

PER SERVING: Calories: 243; Fat: 11g; Carbohydrates: 33g; Phosphorus: 84mg; Potassium: 189mg; Sodium: 145mg; Protein: 4g

MIXED-GRAIN HOT CEREAL

Serves 4/ Prep time: 10 minutes, cook time; 25 minutes

The portion size of this hearty breakfast is quite small, but this cereal, combined with a piece of fruit, will keep you going from morning until lunch. Bulgur wheat is high in fiber, low in fat, and offers a nice nutty taste. Serve this cereal topped with syrup, unsalted butter, or a sprinkle of brown sugar.

Ingredients

2¼ cups water

1¼ cups vanilla rice milk

6 tablespoons uncooked bulgur

2 tablespoons uncooked whole buckwheat

1 cup peeled, sliced apple

6 tablespoons plain uncooked couscous

½ teaspoon ground cinnamon

Directions

1. In a medium saucepan over medium-high heat, heat the water and milk.

2. Bring to a boil, and add the bulgur, buckwheat, and apple.

3. Reduce the heat to low and simmer, stirring occasionally, for 20 to 25 minutes or until the bulgur is tender.

4. Remove the saucepan from the heat and stir in the couscous and cinnamon.

5. Let the saucepan stand, covered, for 10 minutes, then fluff the cereal with a fork before serving.

PER SERVING: Calories: 159; Fat: 1g; Carbohydrates: 34g; Phosphorus: 130mg; Potassium: 116mg; Sodium: 33mg; Protein: 4g

CORN PUDDING

Serves 6/ Prep time: 10 minutes; Cook time: 40 minutes

Corn is a staple food in the United States, and it has been used in every type of dish for centuries. Corn pudding is a classic recipe that has its roots in an English savory custard pudding brought by settlers to New England. The Ener-G baking soda substitute in this recipe, which can be found online as well as in health food stores, it doesn't contain the sodium, potassium, and phosphorus found in regular baking soda.

Ingredients

Unsalted butter, for greasing the baking dish

2 tablespoons all-purpose flour

½ teaspoon Ener-G baking soda substitute

3 eggs

¾ cup unsweetened rice milk, at room temperature

3 tablespoons unsalted butter, melted

2 tablespoons light sour cream

2 tablespoons granulated sugar

2 cups frozen corn kernels, thawed

Directions

1. Preheat the oven to 350°F.

2. Lightly grease an 8-by-8-inch baking dish with butter; set aside.

3. In a small bowl, stir together the flour and baking soda substitute; set aside.

4. In a medium bowl, whisk together the eggs, rice milk, butter, sour cream, and sugar.

5. Stir the flour mixture into the egg mixture until smooth.

6. Add the corn to the batter and stir until very well mixed.

7. Spoon the batter into the baking dish and bake for about 40 minutes or until the pudding is set.

8. Let the pudding cool for about 15 minutes and serve warm.

PER SERVING Calories: 175; Fat: 10g; Carbohydrates: 19g; Phosphorus: 111mg; Potassium: 170mg; Sodium: 62mg; Protein: 5g

RHUBARB BREAD PUDDING

Serves 6/ Prep time: 15 minutes, plus 30 minutes to soak ;Cook time: 50 minutes

In medieval times, bread pudding was peasant food created to use up stale bread. Most dessert bread puddings are quite sweet, but this version is more tart, and would be perfect for a lazy weekend-morning breakfast. Rhubarb is used more like fruit in cooking, but it is actually a vegetable. It is an excellent source of fiber and vitamin C.

Ingredients

Unsalted butter, for greasing the baking dish

1½ cups unsweetened rice milk

3 eggs

½ cup granulated sugar

1 tablespoon cornstarch

1 vanilla bean, split

10 thick pieces white bread, cut into 1-inch chunks

2 cups chopped fresh rhubarb

Directions

1. Preheat the oven to 350°F.

2. Lightly grease an 8-by-8-inch baking dish with butter; set aside.

3. In a large bowl, whisk together the rice milk, eggs, sugar, and cornstarch.

4. Scrape the vanilla seeds into the milk mixture and whisk to blend.

5. Add the bread to the egg mixture and stir to completely coat the bread.

6. Add the chopped rhubarb and stir to combine.

7. Let the bread and egg mixture soak for 30 minutes.

8. Spoon the mixture into the prepared baking dish, cover with aluminum foil, and bake for 40 minutes.

9. Uncover the bread pudding and bake for an additional 10 minutes or until the pudding is golden brown and set.

10. Serve warm.

Dialysis modification: Reduce the rhubarb to 1 cup to bring the potassium to less than 150 mg per serving or remove the rhubarb completly to bring the potassium to less than 75 mg per serving. The bread pudding is delicious without the rhubarb, but it will be less tart.

PER SERVING Calories: 197; Fat: 4g; Carbohydrates: 35g; Phosphorus: 109mg; Potassium: 192mg; Sodium: 159mg; Protein: 6g

CINNAMON-NUTMEG BLUEBERRY MUFFINS

Makes 12 muffins/ Prep time: 15 minutes; Cook time: 30 minutes

Fresh blueberries are the best option for these muffins, because frozen berries can create an unfortunate purple-hued batter and add too much moisture.

Blueberries are an excellent source of vitamin C and other antioxidants, and they are very high in fiber.

Ingredients

2 cups unsweetened rice milk

1 tablespoon apple cider vinegar

3½ cups all-purpose flour

1 cup granulated sugar

1 tablespoon Ener-G baking soda substitute

1 teaspoon ground cinnamon

½ teaspoon ground nutmeg Pinch ground ginger

½ cup canola oil

2 tablespoons pure vanilla extract

2½ cups fresh blueberries

Directions

1. Preheat the oven to 375°F.
2. Line the cups of a muffin pan with paper liners; set aside.
3. In a small bowl, stir together the rice milk and vinegar; set aside for 10 minutes.
4. In a large bowl, stir together the flour, sugar, baking soda substitute, cinnamon, nutmeg, and ginger until well mixed. Add the oil and vanilla to the milk mixture and stir to blend.
5. Add the milk mixture to the dry ingredients and stir until just combined.
6. Fold in the blueberries. Spoon the muffin batter evenly into the cups.
7. Bake the muffins for 25 to 30 minutes or until golden and a toothpick inserted in the center of a muffin comes out clean.
8. Allow the muffins to cool for 15 minutes before serving.

PER SERVING Calories: 331; Fat: 11g; Carbohydrates: 52g; Phosphorus: 90mg; Potassium: 89mg; Sodium: 35mg; Protein: 6g

FRUIT AND CHEESE BREAKFAST WRAP

Serves 2 / Prep time: 10 minutes

If you need to get up and run out the door because of an activity-packed day, this tasty wrap is a perfect choice. If you don't have apples, pears, strawberries, and peaches are also a delicious combination with the tart cheese. These wraps can be made the night before to save even more time.

ingredients

2 (6-inch) flour tortillas

2 tablespoons plain cream cheese

1 apple, peeled, cored, and sliced thin

1 tablespoon honey

Directions

1. Lay both tortillas on a clean work surface and spread 1 tablespoon of cream cheese onto each tortilla, leaving about ½ inch around the edges.

2. Arrange the apple slices on the cream cheese, just off the center of the tortilla on

the side closest to you, leaving about 1½ inches on each side and 2 inches on the bottom.

3. Sprinkle the apples lightly with honey.

4. Fold the left and right edges of the tortillas into the center, laying the edge over the apples.

5. Taking the tortilla edge closest to you, fold it over the fruit and the side pieces. Roll the tortilla away from you, creating a snug wrap.

6. Repeat with the second tortilla.

PER SERVING Calories: 188; Fat: 6g; Carbohydrates: 33g; Phosphorus: 73mg; Potassium: 136mg; Sodium: 177mg; Protein: 4g

EGG-IN-THE-HOLE

Serves 2/ Prep time: 5 minutes;Cook time: 5 minutes

This simple breakfast takes about 5 minutes from fridge to plate and tastes incredibly rich and delicious. The egg white will spread under the butter- browned toasted bread, leaving a perfectly framed yolk. You can top this dish with the chopped herbs of your choice, but chives offer a nice flavor.

ingredients
2 (½-inch-thick) slices Italian bread
¼ cup unsalted butter
2 eggs
2 tablespoons chopped fresh chives
Pinch cayenne pepper Freshly ground black pepper

Directions
1. Using a cookie cutter or a small glass, cut a 2-inch round from the center of each piece of bread.
2. In a large nonstick skillet over medium-high heat, melt the butter.

3. Place the bread in the skillet, toast it for 1 minute, and then flip the bread over.

4. Crack the eggs into the holes the center of the bread and cook for about 2 minutes or until the eggs are set and the bread is golden brown.

5. Top with chopped chives, cayenne pepper, and black pepper.

6. Cook the bread for another 2 minutes.

7. Transfer an egg-in-the-hole to each plate to serve.

PER SERVING Calories: 304; Fat: 29g; Carbohydrates: 12g; Phosphorus: 119mg; Potassium: 109mg; Sodium: 204mg; Protein: 9g

SKILLET-BAKED PANCAKE
Serves 2/Prep time: 15 minutes; Cook time: 20 minutes

If you are used to flat pancakes, the puffy appearance of this pancake might be a surprise when it comes out of the oven. Don't be alarmed if the pancake collapses before you cut it into servings—this is normal. Deflation of the pancake creates a creamy, pudding-like center. You can top this golden beauty with fruit, a drizzle of syrup, or a dollop of whipped topping.

Ingredients
2 eggs
½ cup unsweetened rice milk
½ cup all-purpose flour
¼ teaspoon ground cinnamon Pinch ground nutmeg
Cooking spray, for greasing the skillet

Directions
1. Preheat the oven to 450°F.
2. In a medium bowl, whisk together the eggs and rice milk.

3. Stir in the flour, cinnamon, and nutmeg until blended but still slightly lumpy, but do not overmix.

4. Spray a 9-inch ovenproof skillet with cooking spray and place the skillet in the preheated oven for 5 minutes.

5. Remove the skillet carefully and pour the pancake batter into the skillet.

6. Put back the skillet to the oven and bake the pancake for about 20 minutes or until it is puffed up and crispy on the edges.

7. Cut the pancake into halves to serve.

Dialysis modification: If you need additional protein in this dish, whisk in an extra egg white. There will be no change in texture or taste.

PER SERVING Calories: 161; Fat: 1g; Carbohydrates: 30g; Phosphorus: 73mg; Potassium: 106mg; Sodium: 79mg; Protein: 7g

STRAWBERRY–CREAM CHEESE STUFFED FRENCH TOAST

Serves 4/Prep time: 20 minutes, plus overnight to soak; Cook time: 1 hour, 5 minutes

If you need something out of the ordinary to serve for breakfast or brunch, try this elegant creation. There is no mess or fuss in the morning because the entire recipe can be put together the night before and left to soak in the refrigerator.

The next morning, simply put the baking dish in the oven. In one hour, you can serve a golden, crispy, sweet treat to your family or guests.

Cooking spray, for greasing the baking dish.

Ingredients
½ cup plain cream cheese
4 tablespoons strawberry jam
8 slices thick white bread
2 eggs, beaten
½ cup unsweetened rice milk
1 teaspoon pure vanilla extract
1 tablespoon granulated sugar

¼ teaspoon ground cinnamon

Directions

1. Preheat the oven to 350°F.
2. Spray an 8-by-8-inch baking dish with cooking spray; set aside.
3. In a small bowl, stir together the cream cheese and jam until well blended.
4. Spread 3 tablespoons of the cream cheese mixture onto 4 slices of bread and top with the remaining 4 slices to make sandwiches.
5. In a medium bowl, whisk together the eggs, milk, and vanilla until smooth.
6. Dip the sandwiches into the egg mixture and lay them in the baking dish.
7. Pour any remaining egg mixture over the sandwiches and sprinkle them evenly with sugar and cinnamon.
8. Cover the dish with foil and refrigerate overnight.
9. Bake the French toast, covered, for 1 hour.
10. Remove the foil and bake for 5 minutes more or until the French toast is golden.
11. Serve warm.

PER SERVING Calories: 233; Fat: 9g; Carbohydrates: 30g; Phosphorus: 102mg;

Potassium: 104mg; Sodium: 270mg;
Protein: 9g

SUMMER VEGETABLE OMELET

Serves 3/ Prep time: 15 minutes, cook time: 10 minutes

A good-quality nonstick pan is crucial when making omelets, especially when working with only egg whites. This omelet incorporates one whole egg among the whites, so the omelet will set more easily. The vegetables in the dish can include whatever you have on hand, or you can chop up an assortment of fresh herbs instead.

Ingredients
4 egg whites
1 egg
2 tablespoons chopped fresh parsley
2 tablespoons water
Olive oil spray, for greasing the skillet
½ cup chopped and boiled red bell pepper

¼ cup chopped scallion, both green and white parts Freshly ground black pepper

Directions

1. In a small bowl, whisk together the egg whites, egg, parsley, and water until well blended; set aside.
2. Generously spray a large nonstick skillet with olive oil spray, and place it over medium-high heat.
3. Sauté the peppers and scallion for about 3 minutes or until softened.
4. Pour the egg mixture into the skillet over the vegetables and cook, swirling the skillet, for about 2 minutes or until the edges of the egg start to set.
5. Lift up the set edges and tilt the pan so that the uncooked egg can flow under the cooked egg.
6. Continue lifting and cooking the egg for about 4 minutes or until the omelet is set.
7. Loosen the omelet with a spatula and fold it in half. Cut the folded omelet into 3 portions and transfer the omelets to serving plates.
8. Season with black pepper and serve.

PER SERVING Calories: 77; Fat: 3g; Carbohydrates: 2g; Phosphorus: 67mg;

Potassium: 194mg; Sodium: 229mg; Protein: 12g

CHEESY SCRAMBLED EGGS WITH FRESH HERBS

Serves 4/Prep time: 15 minutes,cook time: 10 minutes

Cream cheese, chopped fresh herbs, and tender chopped scallion elevate humble scrambled eggs to a new culinary level. The cheese will create luscious golden curds that make these eggs seem to melt in your mouth. You can add chopped, cooked chicken or vegetables such as asparagus and red bell pepper if you want a more substantial meal or need to feed more people. Serve on white toast.

Ingredients
3 eggs, at room temperature
2 egg whites, at room temperature
½ cup cream cheese, at room temperature
¼ cup unsweetened rice milk

1 tablespoon finely chopped scallion, green part only
1 tablespoon chopped fresh tarragon
2 tablespoons unsalted butter Freshly ground black pepper

Directions

1. In a medium bowl, whisk together the eggs, egg whites, cream cheese, rice milk, scallions, and tarragon until well blended and smooth.
2. In a large skillet over medium-high heat, melt the butter, swirling to coat the skillet evenly.
3. Pour in the egg mixture and cook, stirring, for about 5 minutes or until the eggs are thick and the curds creamy. Season with pepper.

PER SERVING Calories: 221; Fat: 19g; Carbohydrates: 3g; Phosphorus: 119mg; Potassium: 140mg; Sodium: 193mg; Protein: 8g

EGG AND VEGGIE MUFFINS

Serves 4/ Prep time: 15 minutes, cook time: 20 minutes

These muffins are more like mini crustless quiches, but they bake in muffin pans, so the name fits. You can double the recipe and make enough to freeze for quick, 2-minute microwavable meals later in the week. Egg muffins also can be wrapped in tortillas or stuffed in a pita with shredded lettuce for lunch or a filling snack.

ingredients
Cooking spray, for greasing the muffin pans
4 eggs
2 tablespoons unsweetened rice milk
½ sweet onion, finely chopped
½ red bell pepper, finely chopped
1 tablespoon chopped fresh parsley pinch red pepper flakes
Pinch freshly ground black pepper

Directions
1. Preheat the oven to 350°F.
2. Spray 4 muffin pans with cooking spray; set aside.

3. In a large bowl, whisk together the eggs, milk, onion, red pepper, parsley, red pepper flakes, and black pepper until well combined.

4. Pour the egg mixture into the prepared muffin pans.

5. Bake 18 to 20 minutes or until the muffins are puffed and golden.

6. Serve warm or cold.

PER SERVING Calories: 84; Fat: 5g; Carbohydrates: 3g; Phosphorus: 110mg; Potassium: 117mg; Sodium: 75mg; Protein: 7g

CURRIED EGG PITA POCKETS

Serves 4/ Prep time: 15 minutes; Cook time: 5 minutes

Pitas are handy, portable containers for an assortment of nutritious fillings. Make sure you purchase pita bread that is designed to open up (e.g., Greek-style pitas) because some pitas do not separate easily and are used more as a wrap or flatbread.

Ingredients

3 eggs, beaten

1 scallion, both green and white parts, finely chopped

½ red bell pepper, finely chopped

2 teaspoons unsalted butter

1 teaspoon curry powder

½ teaspoon ground ginger

2 tablespoons light sour cream

2 (4-inch) plain pita bread pockets, halved

½ cup julienned English cucumber

1 cup roughly chopped watercress

Directions

1. In a small bowl, whisk together the eggs, scallion, and red pepper until well blended.

2. In a large nonstick skillet over medium heat, melt the butter.

3. Pour the egg mixture into the skillet and cook for about 3 minutes or until the eggs are just set, swirling the skillet but not stirring. Remove the eggs from the heat; set aside.

4. In a small bowl, stir together the curry powder, ginger, and sour cream until well blended.

5. Divide the curry sauce among the 4 halves of the pita bread, spreading it out on one inside edge.

6. Divide the cucumber and watercress evenly between the halves.

7. Spoon the eggs into the halves, dividing the mixture evenly, to serve.

PER SERVING Calories: 127; Fat: 7g; Carbohydrates: 10g; Phosphorus: 108mg; Potassium: 169mg; Sodium: 139mg; Protein: 7g

ROASTED ONION GARLIC DIP

Serves 6 [¼ cup = 1 serving] Prep time: 15 minutes, plus 1 hour to chill; Cook time: 1 hour

Roasting vegetables removes any bitterness, leaving only a rich, sweet flavor that is fabulous in recipes such as this robust, versatile dish. If the garlic cloves are very young and green, boil them in milk first for 5 minutes, rinse them, and then season the cloves with oil. This process will draw out some of the overwhelmingly sharp garlic taste before roasting. Serve this dip with vegetables or pita triangles.

Ingredients

1 large sweet onion, peeled and cut into eighths
8 garlic cloves
2 teaspoons olive oil
½ cup light sour cream
1 tablespoon fresh lemon juice
1 tablespoon chopped fresh parsley
1 teaspoon chopped fresh thyme
Freshly ground black pepper

Directions

1. Preheat the oven to 425°F.

2. In a small bowl, put the onion and garlic with the olive oil.

3. Transfer the onion and garlic to a piece of aluminum foil and wrap the vegetables loosely in a packet.

4. Place the foil packet on a small baking sheet and place the sheet in the oven.

5. Roast the vegetables for 50 minutes to 1 hour, or until they are very fragrant and golden.

6. Remove the packet from the oven and allow it to cool for 15 minutes.

7. In a medium bowl, stir together the sour cream, lemon juice, parsley, thyme, and black pepper.

8. Open the foil packet carefully and transfer the vegetables to a cutting board.

9. Chop the vegetables and add them to the sour cream mixture. Stir to combine.

10. Cover the dip and chill in the refrigerator for 1 hour before serving.

PER SERVING Calories: 44; Fat: 3g; Carbohydrates: 5g; Phosphorus: 22mg; Potassium: 79mg; Sodium: 10mg; Protein: 1g

BABA GHANOUSH

Serves 6/ Prep time: 20 minutes; Cook time: 30 minutes

Baba ghanoush is a dip that is similar to hummus, but eggplant is the star attraction. Eggplant can get very oily when it is cooked because it soaks up fat like a sponge, so make sure to brush it lightly with oil. You also can make a double batch of this recipe and use a couple of spoonfuls as an easy pasta sauce.

Ingredients

1 medium eggplant, halved and scored with a crosshatch pattern on the cut sides
1 tablespoon olive oil, plus extra for brushing
1 large sweet onion, peeled and diced
2 garlic cloves, halved
1 teaspoon ground cumin
1 teaspoon ground coriander
1 tablespoon lemon juice
Freshly ground black pepper

Directions

1. Preheat the oven to 400°F.

2. Line 2 baking sheets with parchment paper.

3 Brush the eggplant halves with olive oil and place them, cut-side down, on 1 baking sheet.

4. In a small bowl, mix together the onion, garlic, 1 tablespoon olive oil, cumin, and coriander.

5. Spread the seasoned onions on the other baking sheet.

6. Place both baking sheets in the oven and roast the onions for about 20 minutes and the eggplant for 30 minutes, or until softened and browned.

7. Remove the vegetables from the oven and scrape the eggplant flesh into a bowl.

8. Transfer the onions and garlic to a cutting board and chop coarsely; add to the eggplant.

9. Stir in the lemon juice and pepper.

10. Serve warm or chilled.

PER SERVING Calories: 45; Fat: 2g; Carbohydrates: 6g; Phosphorus: 23mg; Potassium: 195mg; Sodium: 3mg; Protein: 1g

CHEESE-HERB DIP

Serves 8 [3 tablespoons = 1 serving]
Prep time: 20 minutes

An easy, never-fails-to-please dip is a valuable addition to your culinary toolbox. If you are attending a neighborhood block party, having guests, or for a family event, or you want something delicious on hand for movie night at home, this dip is a perfect choice. A bit of finely chopped vegetables or jalapeño peppers would also work with the base ingredients, so feel free to experiment with the recipe. Serve with cut vegetables.

Ingredients

1 cup cream cheese
½ cup unsweetened rice milk
½ scallion, green part only, finely chopped
1 tablespoon chopped fresh parsley
1 tablespoon chopped fresh basil
1 tablespoon freshly squeezed lemon juice
1 teaspoon minced garlic
½ teaspoon chopped fresh thyme
¼ teaspoon freshly ground black pepper

Directions

1. In a medium bowl, mix together the cream cheese, milk, scallion, parsley, basil, lemon juice, garlic, thyme, and pepper until well combined.

2. Store the dip in a sealed container in the refrigerator for up to 1 week.

PER SERVING Calories: 108; Fat: 10g; Carbohydrates: 3g; Phosphorus: 40mg; Potassium: 52mg; Sodium: 112mg; Protein: 2g

SPICY KALE CHIPS

Serves 6/Prep time: 20 minutes; Cook time: 25 minutes

Kale has become a phenomenon in the last few decades, going from a food eaten only by health fanatics to a mainstream grocery item consumed by just about everyone. Kale chips are surprisingly crunchy, richly flavored, and are best eaten immediately if you are making your own. The trick to crispy chips is to leaves the kale to very thoroughly dry and make sure the oil is massaged evenly into every leaf before baking.

Ingredients
2 cups kale
2 teaspoons olive oil
¼ teaspoon chili powder Pinch cayenne pepper

Directions
1. Preheat the oven to 300°F.
2. Line 2 baking sheets with parchment paper; set aside.
3. Remove the stems from the kale and tear the leaves into 2-inch pieces.
4. Wash the kale and dry it completely.
5. Transfer the kale to a large bowl and drizzle with olive oil.
6. Use your hands to toss the kale with the oil, taking care to coat each leaf evenly.
7. Season the kale with chili powder and cayenne pepper and toss to combine thoroughly.
8. Spread the seasoned kale in a single layer on each baking sheet. Do not overlap the leaves.

9. Bake the kale, rotating the pans once, for 20 to 25 minutes or until it is crisp and dry.

10. Remove the trays from the oven and allow the chips to cool on the trays for 5 minutes.

11. Serve immediately.

PER SERVING Calories: 24; Fat: 2g; Carbohydrates: 2g; Phosphorus: 21mg; Potassium: 111mg; Sodium: ; Protein: 1g

CINNAMON TORTILLA CHIPS

Serves 6/ Prep time: 15 minutes; Cook time: 10 minutes

Cinnamon adds spice to savory and sweet dishes in a variety of different kind of cooking. Ground cinnamon comes from the bark of the cinnamon tree.

Cinnamon may play a role in treating and healing chronic wounds because of the essential oils found in the bark. It also may help improve blood sugar and cholesterol levels in people with type 2 diabetes.

Ingredients

2 teaspoons granulated sugar

½ teaspoon ground cinnamon Pinch ground nutmeg

3 (6-inch) flour tortillas

Cooking spray, for coating the tortillas

Directions

1. Preheat the oven to 350°F.

2. Line a baking sheet with parchment paper.

3. In a small bowl, stir together the sugar, cinnamon, and nutmeg.

4. Lay the tortillas on a clean work surface and spray both sides of each lightly with cooking spray.

5. Sprinkle the cinnamon sugar evenly over both sides of each tortilla.

6. Cut the tortillas into 16 wedges each and place them on the baking sheet.

7. Bake the tortilla wedges, turning once, for about 10 minutes or until crisp.

8. Cool the chips and store in a sealed container at room temperature for up to 1 week.

PER SERVING Calories: 51; Fat: 1g; Carbohydrates: 9g; Phosphorus: 29mg;

Potassium: 24mg; Sodium: 103mg; Protein: 1g

SWEET AND SPICY KETTLE CORN

Serves 8/ Prep time: 1 minute; Cook time: 5 minutes

Microwave popcorn is an incredibly popular snack, but its ingredients and cooking process have caused preoccupation in recent years. This recipe uses an old-fashioned stove-top technique that allows you to add the ingredients and flavorings you want. Take care not to allow the pot to get too hot, or the sugar will burn instead of caramelize.

Ingrediemts
3 tablespoons olive oil
1 cup popcorn kernels
½ cup brown sugar Pinch cayenne pepper

Directions

1. Place a large pot with lid over medium heat and add the olive oil with a few popcorn kernels.

2. Shake the pot lightly until the popcorn kernels pop. Add the rest of the kernels and sugar to the pot.

3. Pop the kernels with the lid on the pot, shaking constantly, until they are all popped.

4. Remove the pot from the heat and transfer the popcorn to a large bowl.

5. Toss the popcorn with the cayenne pepper and serve.

PER SERVING Calories: 186; Fat: 6g; Carbohydrates: 30g; Phosphorus: 85mg; Potassium: 90mg; Sodium: 5mg; Protein: 3g

BLUEBERRIES AND CREAM ICE POPS
Makes 6 pops / Prep time: 10 minutes, plus 3 hours to freeze

Ice pops are a cheerful treat. They evoke memories of sunny childhood summers spent licking ice pops that dripped down your hand and your scuffed sneakers.

You can use any type of fruit, such as strawberries, raspberries, peaches, and watermelon, for the base.

Ingredients
3 cups fresh blueberries

1 teaspoon freshly squeezed lemon juice

¼ cup unsweetened rice milk

¼ cup light sour cream

¼ cup granulated sugar

½ teaspoon pure vanilla extract

¼ teaspoon ground cinnamon

Directions

1. Put the blueberries, lemon juice, rice milk, sour cream, sugar, vanilla, and cinnamon in a blender and purée until smooth.

2. Spoon the mixture into ice-pop molds and freeze for 3 to 4 hours or until very firm.

PER SERVING Calories: 78; Fat: 1g; Carbohydrates: 18g; Phosphorus: 20mg; Potassium: 55mg; Sodium: 12mg; Protein: 1g

CANDIED GINGER ICE MILK

Makes 4 cups/Prep time: 20 minutes, plus 1 hour to freeze; Cook time: 15 minutes

Ice milk is a refreshing version of ice cream, and you will only need a small portion of this cool treat to satisfy your taste buds. If you do not have an ice- cream maker, pour the mixture in a metal baking pan and place it in the freezer. Stir, and then scrape, the liquid as it freezes, creating an ice cream–like texture.

Ingredients
4 cups vanilla rice milk
½ cup granulated sugar
1 (4-inch) piece fresh ginger, peeled and sliced thin
¼ teaspoon ground nutmeg
¼ cup finely chopped candied ginger

Directions

1. In a large saucepan over medium heat, stir together the milk, sugar, and fresh ginger.

2. Heat the milk mixture, stirring occasionally, for about 5 minutes or until it is almost boiling.

3. Turn down the heat to low and simmer for 15 minutes.

4. Remove the milk mixture from the heat and add the ground nutmeg. Let the mixture sit for 1 hour to infuse the flavor.

5. Strain the milk mixture through a fine sieve into a medium bowl to remove the ginger.

6. Add the candied ginger, and place the mixture in the refrigerator to chill completely.

7. Freeze the ginger ice in an ice-cream maker according to the manufacturer's instructions.

8. Store the finished treat in the freezer in a sealed container for up to 3 months.

PER SERVING Calories: 108; Fat: 1g; Carbohydrates: 24g; Phosphorus: 68mg; Potassium: 45mg; Sodium: 47mg; Protein: 0g

MERINGUE COOKIES

**Makes 24 cookies/ Prep time: 30 minutes
Cook time: 30 minutes**

Meringue cookies have a history that stretches back in the centuries. They appear in a French document from 1604, as well as in antique cookbooks in other countries. This recipe is a basic French meringue that does not require the candy thermometer or bain-marie needed in the Italian and Swiss versions. Make sure your egg whites are completely yolk-free or they will not whip up to the right texture and height. Also, your whisk or beaters need to be completely free of fat.

Ingredients

4 egg whites, at room temperature

1 cup granulated sugar

1 teaspoon pure vanilla extract

1 teaspoon almond extract

Directions

1. Preheat the oven to 300°F.

2. Line 2 baking sheets with parchment; set aside.

3. In a large stainless steel bowl, beat the egg whites until stiff peaks form.

4. Add the granulated sugar 1 tablespoon at a time, beating well to incorporate after each addition, until all the sugar is used and the meringue is thick and glossy.

5. Beat in the vanilla extract and almond extract.

6. Using a tablespoon, drop the meringue batter onto the baking sheets, spacing the cookies evenly.

7. Bake the cookies for about 30 minutes or until they are crisp.

8. Remove the cookies from the oven and let them cool on wire racks.

9. Store the cookies in an airtight container at room temperature for up to 1 week.

PER SERVING Calories: 36; Fat: 0g; Carbohydrates: 8g; Phosphorus: 1mg; Potassium: 10mg; Sodium: 9mg; Protein: 1g

CORNBREAD

Serves 10/ Prep time: 10 minutes; Cook time: 20 minutes

Sometimes people think that corn bread is unhealthy because many chefs and home cooks add fat-and sodium-laden ingredients such as bacon and heaps of cheese. This recipe has all the buttery, sweet flavor of traditional corn bread without the unhealthy additions. You can add chopped jalapeño pepper or bits of roasted red bell pepper for a different, more complex taste.

Ingredients

Cooking spray, for greasing the baking dish

1¼ cups yellow cornmeal

¾ cup all-purpose flour

1 tablespoon Ener-G baking soda substitute

½ cup granulated sugar

 2 eggs

1 cup unsweetened, unfortified rice milk

2 tablespoons olive oil

Procedure

1. Preheat the oven to 425°F.

2. Lightly spray an 8-by-8-inch baking dish with cooking spray; set aside.

3. In a medium bowl, stir together the cornmeal, flour, baking soda substitute, and sugar.

4. In a small bowl, whisk together the eggs, rice milk, and olive oil until blended.

5. Add the wet ingredients to the dry ingredients and stir until well combined.

6. Pour the batter into the baking dish and bake for about 20 minutes or until golden and cooked through.

7. Serve warm.

PER SERVING Calories: 198; Fat: 5g; Carbohydrates: 34g; Phosphorus: 88mg; Potassium: 94mg; Sodium: 25mg; Protein: 4g

ROASTED RED PEPPER AND CHICKEN CROSTINI

Serves 4/ Prep time: 10 minutes; Cook time: 5 minutes

Crostini and bruschetta are similar, but bruschetta usually has vegetable-or fruit-based toppings and crostini can be also topped with meats, fish, or poultry. The best crostini are made with bread that has been brushed with olive oil and grilled, so if you want to fire up your barbecue to create this recipe, the results will be spectacular. Make sure you grill both sides for the perfect crunch.

Ingredients

2 tablespoons olive oil

½ teaspoon minced garlic

4 slices French bread

1 roasted red bell pepper, chopped

4 ounces cooked chicken breast, shredded

½ cup chopped fresh basil

Directions

1. Preheat the oven to 400°F.

2. Line a baking sheet with aluminum foil.

3. In a small bowl, mix together the olive oil and garlic.

4. Brush both sides of each piece of bread with the olive oil mixture.

5. Place the bread on the baking sheet and toast in the oven, turning once, for about 5 minutes or until both sides are golden and crisp.

6. In a medium bowl, stir together the red pepper, chicken, and basil.

7. Top each toasted bread slice with the red pepper mixture and serve.

PER SERVING Calories: 184; Fat: 8g; Carbohydrates: 19g; Phosphorus: 87mg; Potassium: 152mg; Sodium: 175mg; Protein: 9g

CUCUMBER-WRAPPED VEGETABLE ROLLS

Serves 8 / Prep time: 30 minutes

Create the perfect vegetable-wrapped roll hinges on the correct thinness of the vegetable you use as a wrapper. Cutting thin cucumber strips is much easier if you use a peeler, cheese cutter, or mandoline. A mandoline is a kitchen tool that slices very thin strips, makes batons, and cuts a pretty crosshatch using parallel and perpendicular blades. If you prepare a lot of fruits or vegetables, a mandoline is a smart investment.

Ingredients

½ cup finely shredded red cabbage

½ cup grated carrot

¼ cup julienned red bell pepper

¼ cup julienned scallion, both green and white parts

¼ cup chopped cilantro

1 tablespoon olive oil

¼ teaspoon ground cumin

¼ teaspoon freshly ground black pepper

1 English cucumber, sliced into 8 very thin strips with a vegetable peeler

Directions

1. In a medium bowl, toss together the cabbage, carrot, red pepper, scallion, cilantro, olive oil, cumin, and black pepper until well mixed.

2. Divide the vegetable filling among the cucumber strips, placing the filling close to one end of the strip.

3. Roll up the cucumber strips around the filling and secure with a wooden pick.

4. Repeat with each cucumber strip.

PER SERVING Calories: 26; Fat: 2g; Carbohydrates: 3g; Phosphorus: 14mg; Potassium: 95mg; Sodium: 7mg; Protein: 0g

ANTOJITOS

Serves 8 / Prep time: 20 minutes

Antojitos, loosely translated, means "little cravings," which is accurate because these tempting spirals are addictive. The ingredients vary regionally, highlighting local cheeses, meats, and vegetables. These snacks are also called botanas in the Yucatán Peninsula. Although often the are served cold, you can melt the cheese under the broiler.

Ingredients
6 ounces plain cream cheese, at room temperature
½ jalapeño pepper, finely chopped
½ scallion, green part only, chopped
¼ cup finely chopped red bell pepper
½ teaspoon ground cumin
½ teaspoon ground coriander
½ teaspoon chili powder 3 (8-inch) flour tortillas

Directions

1. In a medium bowl, mix together the cream cheese, jalapeño pepper, scallion, red bell pepper, cumin, coriander, and chili powder until well blended.

2. Divide the cream cheese mixture evenly among the 3 tortillas, spreading the cheese in a thin layer and leaving a ¼-inch edge all the way around.

3. Roll the tortillas like a jelly roll and wrap each tightly in plastic wrap.

4. Refrigerate the rolls for about 1 hour or until they are set.

5. Cut the tortilla rolls into 1-inch pieces and arrange them on a plate to serve.

PER SERVING Calories: 110; Fat: 8g; Carbohydrates: 7g; Phosphorus: 47mg; Potassium: 72mg; Sodium: 215mg; Protein: 2g

CHICKEN-VEGETABLE KEBABS

Serves 4/Prep time: 15 minutes, plus 1 hour to marinate; Cook time: 12 minutes

These colorful kebabs are not meant to be anything more than a snack, so if you want to eat them as a meal, you have to eat more than one. The onion can be tricky to get on the skewer as wedges, so you may want to use pearl onions. These little onions will fit perfectly on the skewer without separating into layers.

Ingredients

2 tablespoons olive oil
2 tablespoons freshly squeezed lemon juice
½ teaspoon minced garlic
½ teaspoon chopped fresh thyme
4 ounces boneless, skinless chicken breast, cut into 8 pieces
1 small summer squash, cut into 8 pieces
½ medium onion, cut into 8 pieces

Directions

1. In a medium bowl, stir together the olive oil, lemon juice, garlic, and thyme.

2. Add the chicken to the bowl and stir to coat.

3. Cover the bowl with plastic wrap and place the chicken in the refrigerator to marinate for 1 hour.

4. Thread the squash, onion, and chicken pieces onto 4 large skewers, evenly dividing the vegetables and meat among the skewers.

5. Heat a barbecue to medium and grill the skewers, turning at least 2 times, for 10 to 12 minutes or until the chicken is cooked through.

PER SERVING Calories: 106; Fat: 8g; Carbohydrates: 3g; Phosphorus: 77mg; Potassium: 199mg; Sodium: 14mg; Protein: 7g

FIVE-SPICE CHICKEN LETTUCE WRAPS
Serves 8 / Prep time: 30 minutes

Lettuce wraps are a common street food in Asia, filled with exotic ingredients and spices. Boston lettuce leaves are the best choice for the wrap part of the recipe because they are thin and do not have a stiff rib down the center. Green or red-leaf lettuce also works well if you use the outer leaves.

Ingredients
6 ounces cooked chicken breast, minced
1 scallion, both green and white parts, chopped
½ red apple, cored and chopped
½ cup bean sprouts
¼ English cucumber, finely chopped Juice of 1 lime
Zest of 1 lime
2 tablespoons chopped fresh cilantro
½ teaspoon Chinese five-spice powder
8 Boston lettuce leaves

Directions

1. In a large bowl, mix together the chicken, scallions, apple, bean sprouts, cucumber, lime juice, lime zest, cilantro, and five-spice powder.

2. Spoon the chicken mixture evenly among the 8 lettuce leaves.

3. Wrap the lettuce around the chicken mixture and serve.

PER SERVING Calories: 51; Fat: 2g; Carbohydrates: 2g; Phosphorus: 56mg; Potassium: 110mg; Sodium: 16mg; Protein: 7g

SOUPS AND STEW RECIPES

FRENCH ONION SOUP

Serves 4/Prep time: 20 minutes; Cook time: 50 minutes

Creating a perfect French onion soup is a matter of pride for professional chefs, and the proper technique is the topic of heated arguments. The need to caramelize the onions is the only point that is agreed upon by most chefs, so try to dedicate adequate time to this step in this recipe. If your onions are very young and full of liquid, caramelization might need to be helped along by a tablespoon of granulated sugar.

Ingredients

2 tablespoons unsalted butter

4 Vidalia onions, sliced thin

2 cups Easy Chicken Stock (here)

2 cups water

1 tablespoon chopped fresh thyme Freshly ground black pepper

Directions

1. In a large saucepan over medium heat, melt the butter.

2. Add the onions to the saucepan and cook them slowly, stirring frequently, for about 30 minutes or until the onions are caramelized and tender.

3. Add the chicken stock and water, and bring the soup to a boil.

4. Reduce the heat to low and simmer the soup for 15 minutes.

5. Stir in the thyme and season the soup with pepper.

6. Serve piping hot.

PER SERVING Calories: 90; Fat: 6g; Carbohydrates: 7g; Phosphorus: 22mg; Potassium: 192mg; Sodium: 57mg; Protein: 2g

CREAM OF WATERCRESS SOUP

Serves 4 /Prep time: 15 minutes Cook time: 1 hour, 10 minutes

The gorgeous pastel color of this elegant soup and the lush accent flavor of roasted garlic make this dish a perfect recipe for company. You can certainly make it for a simple family meal, but set the table with fine china and heavy silverware to do the soup justice.

Ingredients
6 garlic cloves
½ teaspoon olive oil
1 teaspoon unsalted butter
½ sweet onion, chopped
4 cups chopped watercress
¼ cup chopped fresh parsley
3 cups water
¼ cup heavy cream
1 tablespoon freshly squeezed lemon juice
Freshly ground black pepper

Directions
1. Preheat the oven to 400°F.
2. Place the garlic on a piece of aluminum foil. Drizzle with olive oil and fold the foil

into a little packet. Place the packet in a pie plate and roast the garlic for about 20 minutes or until very soft.

3. Remove the garlic from the oven; set aside to cool.

4. In a large saucepan over medium-high heat, melt the butter. Sauté the onion for about 4 minutes. Add the watercress and parsley; sauté 5 minutes.

5. Stir in the water and roasted garlic pulp. Bring the soup to a boil, then reduce the heat to low.

6. Simmer the soup for about 20 minutes or until the vegetables are soft.

7. Cool the soup for about 5 minutes, then purée in batches in a food processor (or use a large bowl and a handheld immersion blender), along with the heavy cream.

8. Transfer the soup to the pot, and set over low heat until warmed through.

9. Add the lemon juice and season with pepper.

PER SERVING Calories: 97; Fat: 8g; Carbohydrates: 5g; Phosphorus: 46mg; Potassium: 198mg; Sodium: 23mg; Protein: 2g

CURRIED CAULIFLOWER SOUP

Serves 6/ Prep time: 20 minutes Cook time: 30 minutes

Cauliflower is a cruciferous vegetable that is often used to provide bulk and texture to recipes. This vegetable also soaks up flavors easily, so it is a logical choice for a curried soup. Cauliflower is full of antioxidants, fiber, and B vitamins, and offers many health benefits, including decreasing the risk of cancer, heart disease, and other inflammatory diseases.

ingredients

1 teaspoon unsalted butter

1 small sweet onion, chopped

2 teaspoons minced garlic

1 small head cauliflower, cut into small florets

3 cups water, or more to cover the cauliflower

2 teaspoons curry powder

½ cup light sour cream

3 tablespoons chopped fresh cilantro

Directions

1. In a large saucepan, heat the butter over medium-high heat and sauté the onion and garlic for about 3 minutes or until softened.

2. Add the cauliflower, water, and curry powder.

3. Bring the soup to a boil, then reduce the heat to low and simmer for about 20 minutes or until the cauliflower is tender.

4. Pour the soup into a food processor and purée until the soup is smooth and creamy (or use a large bowl and a handheld immersion blender).

5. Transfer the soup back into a saucepan and stir in the sour cream and cilantro.

6. Heat the soup on medium-low for about 5 minutes or until warmed through.

PER SERVING Calories: 33; Fat: 2g; Carbohydrates: 4g; Phosphorus: 30mg; Potassium: 167mg; Sodium: 22mg; Protein: 1g

ROASTED RED PEPPER AND EGGPLANT SOUP

Serves 6/Prep time: 20 minutes; Cook time: 40 minutes

The process to create this soup may seem odd to you at first, but the results are delightful. Roast the vegetables first and then create the desired soup thickness by blending the finished vegetables with chicken stock. Use homemade chicken stock in your recipes or a carefully vetted commercial product to avoid consuming too much potassium and sodium.

Ingredients

1 small sweet onion, cut into quarters
2 small red bell peppers, halved
2 cups cubed eggplant
2 garlic cloves, crushed
1 tablespoon olive oil
1 cup Easy Chicken Stock (here) Water
¼ cup chopped fresh basil
Freshly ground black pepper

Directions

1. Preheat the oven to 350°F.
2. Put the onions, red peppers, eggplant, and garlic in a large ovenproof baking dish.

3. Drizzle the vegetables with the olive oil.

4. Roast the vegetables for about 30 minutes or until they are slightly charred and soft.

5. Cool the vegetables slightly and remove the skin from the peppers.

6. Purée the vegetables in batches in a food processor (or in a large bowl, using a handheld immersion blender) with the chicken stock.

7. Transfer the soup to a medium pot and add enough water to reach the desired thickness. Heat the soup to a simmer and add the basil.

8. Season with pepper and serve.

PER SERVING Calories: 61; Fat: 2g; Carbohydrates: 9g; Phosphorus: 33mg; Potassium: 198mg; Sodium: 95mg; Protein: 2g

TRADITIONAL CHICKEN-VEGETABLE SOUP

Serves 6/Prep time: 20 minutes; Cook time: 35 minutes

This classic cure for the common cold is a staple soup in many homes. Almost any ingredient works well with this basic recipe, and it freezes well, so make a double batch when you want an easy meal. If you are going to freeze the soup, omit the green beans until the soup is thawed and reheated, or they will end up looking grayish and limp.

Ingredients

1 tablespoon unsalted butter
½ sweet onion, diced
2 teaspoons minced garlic
2 celery stalks, chopped
1 carrot, diced
2 cups chopped cooked chicken breast
1 cup Easy Chicken Stock (here)
4 cups water
1 teaspoon chopped fresh thyme Freshly ground black pepper
2 tablespoons chopped fresh parsley

Directions

1. In a large pot over medium heat, melt the butter.

2. Sauté the onion and garlic for about 3 minutes.

3. Add the celery, carrot, chicken, chicken stock, and water.

4. Bring the soup to a boil, reduce the heat, and simmer for about 30 minutes or until the vegetables are tender.

5. Add the thyme; simmer the soup for 2 minutes.

6. Season with pepper and serve topped with parsley.

PER SERVING Calories: 121; Fat: 6g; Carbohydrates: 2g; Phosphorus: 108mg; Potassium: 199mg; Sodium: 62mg; Protein: 15g

TURKEY-BULGUR SOUP

Serves 6/Prep time: 25 minutes; Cook time: 45 minutes

Turkey may be an overlooked ingredient because chicken seems more available in stores. Turkey is a wonderful, healthy choice for this soup because it is high in protein, zinc, and iron and low in saturated fat. Try to purchase organic, pasture-raised turkey when possible.

Ingredients

1 teaspoon olive oil
½ pound cooked ground turkey, 93% lean
½ sweet onion, chopped
1 teaspoon minced garlic
4 cups water
1 cup Easy Chicken Stock (here)
1 celery stalk, chopped
1 carrot, sliced thin
½ cup shredded green cabbage
½ cup bulgur
2 dried bay leaves
2 tablespoons chopped fresh parsley
1 teaspoon chopped fresh sage
1 teaspoon chopped fresh thyme

Pinch red pepper flakes Freshly ground black pepper

Directions

1. Place a large saucepan over medium-high heat and add the olive oil. Sauté the turkey for about 5 minutes or until the meat is cooked through.

2. Add the onion and garlic and sauté for about 3 minutes or until the vegetables are softened. Add the water, chicken stock, celery, carrot, cabbage, bulgur, and bay leaves.

3. Bring the soup to a boil and then reduce the heat to low and simmer for about 35 minutes or until the bulgur and vegetables are tender.

4. Remove the bay leaves and stir in the parsley, sage, thyme, and red pepper flakes.

5. Season with pepper and serve.

PER SERVING Calories: 77; Fat: 4g; Carbohydrates: 2g; Phosphorus: 82mg; Potassium: 175mg; Sodium: 54mg; Protein: 8g

GROUND BEEF AND RICE SOUP

Serves 6/Prep time: 15 minutes; Cook time: 40 minutes

Try not to break up the ground beef completely when cooking because chunks create a nice texture. For an interesting variation, mix the ground beef with a few tablespoons of bread crumbs, garlic powder, and thyme, and roll the mixture into small meatballs. When the soup is simmering, drop in the meatballs and simmer for about 30 minutes, until they are cooked through.

Ingredients

½ pound extra-lean ground beef
½ small sweet onion, chopped
1 teaspoon minced garlic
2 cups water
1 cup homemade low-sodium beef broth
½ cup long-grain white rice, uncooked
1 celery stalk, chopped
½ cup fresh green beans, cut into 1-inch pieces
1 teaspoon chopped fresh thyme Freshly ground black pepper

Directions

1. Place a large saucepan over medium-high heat and add the ground beef.

2. Sauté, stirring often, for about 6 minutes or until the beef is completely browned.

3. Drain off the excess fat and add the onion and garlic to the saucepan.

4. Sauté the vegetables for about 3 minutes or until they are softened.

5. Add the water, beef broth, rice, and celery.

6. Bring the soup to a boil, reduce the heat to low, and simmer for about 30 minutes or until the rice is tender.

7. Add the green beans and thyme and simmer for 3 minutes.

8. Remove the soup from the heat and season with pepper.

PER SERVING Calories: 154; Fat: 7g; Carbohydrates: 14g; Phosphorus: 76mg; Potassium: 179mg; Sodium: 133mg; Protein: 9g

HERBED CABBAGE STEW

Serves 6/ Prep time: 20 minutes; Cook time: 35 minutes

Cabbage stew is a rustic, filling, low-calorie dish that takes little time to make and gets better while sitting in the refrigerator. This recipe produces a pretty green-hued stew with a herb broth. The cabbage will soften and soak up the flavors, so add a little splash of hot sauce or a spoon of pesto for bolder flavor.

Ingredients
1 teaspoon unsalted butter
½ large sweet onion, chopped
1 teaspoon minced garlic
6 cups shredded green cabbage
3 celery stalks, chopped with the leafy tops
1 scallion, both green and white parts, chopped
2 tablespoons chopped fresh parsley
2 tablespoons freshly squeezed lemon juice
1 tablespoon chopped fresh thyme
1 teaspoon chopped savory
1 teaspoon chopped fresh oregano Water
1 cup fresh green beans, cut into 1-inch pieces Freshly ground black pepper

Directions

1. In a medium stockpot over medium-high heat, melt the butter.

2. Sauté the onion and garlic in the melted butter for about 3 minutes or until the vegetables are softened.

3. Add the cabbage, celery, scallion, parsley, lemon juice, thyme, savory, and oregano to the pot, and add enough water to cover the vegetables by about 4 inches.

4. Bring the soup to a boil, reduce the heat to low, and simmer the soup for about 25 minutes or until the vegetables are tender.

5. Add the green beans and simmer 3 minutes.

6. Season with pepper.

PER SERVING Calories: 33; Fat: 1g; Carbohydrates: 6g; Phosphorus: 29mg; Potassium: 187mg; Sodium: 20mg; Protein: 1g

WINTER CHICKEN STEW

Serves 6 Prep time: 20 minutes; Cook time: 50 minutes

Stew is comfort food you may enjoy most during the cold winter, but you can certainly enjoy this stew in other seasons, too. If you prefer, make it in a slow cooker set on low for 10 hours. Simply brown the chicken breast and add it to all the other ingredients, except the cornstarch, in the slow cooker. Stir in the cornstarch when the stew is done if you need to thicken the sauce.

Ingredients

1 tablespoon olive oil

1 pound boneless, skinless chicken thighs, cut into 1-inch cubes

½ sweet onion, chopped

1 tablespoon minced garlic

2 cups Easy Chicken Stock (here)

2 tablespoons water

1 carrot, sliced

2 celery stalks, sliced

1 turnip, sliced thin

1 tablespoon chopped fresh thyme

1 teaspoon finely chopped fresh rosemary

2 teaspoons cornstarch

Freshly ground black pepper

Directions
1. Put a large saucepan on medium-high heat and add the olive oil.
2. Sauté the chicken for about 6 minutes or until it is lightly browned, stirring often.
3. Add the onion and garlic and sauté for 3 minutes.
4. Add the chicken stock, 1 cup water, carrot, celery, and turnip and bring the stew to a boil.
5. Reduce the heat to low and simmer for about 30 minutes or until the chicken is cooked through and tender.
6. Add the thyme and rosemary and simmer for 3 more minutes.
7. In a small bowl, stir together the 2 tablespoons water and the cornstarch and add the mixture to the stew.
8. Stir to incorporate the cornstarch mixture and cook for 3 to 4 minutes or until the stew thickens.
9. Remove from the heat and season with pepper.

PER SERVING Calories: 141; Fat: 8g; Carbohydrates: 5g; Phosphorus: 53mg;

Potassium: 192mg;   Sodium: 214mg;
Protein: 9g

ROASTED BEEF STEW

Serves 6/ Prep time: 30 minutes; Cook time: 1 hour, 15 minutes

Stew is a very economical dish because it uses cuts of beef less expensive. These cheap cuts are tougher but very flavorful, and they benefit from long cooking times. Roasting the stew in the oven provides the perfect moist environment and timing to produce fork-tender meat.

Ingredients
¼ cup all-purpose flour
1 teaspoon freshly ground black pepper, plus extra for seasoning Pinch cayenne pepper
½ pound boneless beef chuck roast, trimmed of fat and cut into 1-inch chunks
2 tablespoons olive oil
½ sweet onion, chopped
2 teaspoons minced garlic
1 cup homemade beef stock

1 cup plus

2 tablespoons water

1 carrot, cut into ½-inch chunks

2 celery stalks, chopped with greens

1 teaspoon chopped fresh thyme

1 teaspoon cornstarch

2 tablespoons chopped fresh parsley

Directions

1. Preheat the oven to 350°F.

2. Put the flour, black pepper, and cayenne pepper in a large plastic freezer bag and toss to mix.

3. Add the beef chunks to the bag and toss to coat.

4. In a large ovenproof pot, heat the olive oil.

5. Sauté the beef chunks for about 5 minutes or until they are lightly browned. Remove the beef from the pot and set aside on a plate.

6. Add the onion and garlic to the pot and sauté for 3 minutes.

7. Stir in the beef stock and deglaze the pot, scraping up any bits on the bottom.

8. Add 1 cup water, the beef drippings on the plate, the carrot, celery, and thyme.

9. Cover the pot tightly with a lid or aluminum foil and place in the oven.

10. Bake the stew, stirring occasionally, for about 1 hour or until the meat is very tender.

11. Remove the stew from the oven.

12. In a small bowl, stir together the 2 tablespoons water and the cornstarch and then stir the mixture into the hot stew to thicken the sauce.

13. Season the stew with black pepper and serve topped with parsley.

PER SERVING Calories: 163; Fat: 10g; Carbohydrates: 7g; Phosphorus: 89mg; Potassium: 200mg; Sodium: 121mg; Protein: 11g

SALADS RECIPES

LEAF LETTUCE AND CARROT SALAD WITH BALSAMIC VINAIGRETTE

Serves 4 / Prep time: 25 minutes

A simple salad combined with flavorful vinaigrette is a wonderful starter or light meal when topped with a piece of broiled fish or grilled chicken. You can easily make more of the vinaigrette then the recipe suggest if you want to keep some dressing on hand. Add all the vinaigrette ingredients to a mason jar and shake it up whenever you need it.

Ingredients
FOR THE VINAIGRETTE
½ cup olive oil
4 tablespoons balsamic vinegar
2 tablespoons chopped fresh oregano Pinch red pepper flakes
Freshly ground black pepper

FOR THE SALAD

4 cups shredded green leaf lettuce 1 carrot, shredded

¾ cup fresh green beans, cut into 1-inch pieces

3 large radishes, sliced thin

Directions

TO MAKE THE VINAIGRETTE

1. In a small bowl, whisk together the olive oil, balsamic vinegar, oregano, and red pepper flakes.

2. Season with pepper.

TO MAKE THE SALAD

1. In a large bowl, toss together the lettuce, carrot, green beans, and radishes.

2. Add the vinaigrette to the vegetables and toss to coat.

3. Arrange the salad on 4 plates to serve.

PER SERVING Calories: 273; Fat: 27g; Carbohydrates: 7g; Phosphorus: 30mg; Potassium: 197mg; Sodium: 27mg; Protein: 1g

STRAWBERRY-WATERCRESS SALAD WITH ALMOND DRESSING

Serves 6 / Prep time: 15 minutes

Fresh, ripe strawberries add a splash of vivid color and sweetness to this salad, and the almond dressing is an unexpected twist. Strawberries are packed with nutrients—they are an excellent source of vitamin C, folate, and fiber, and they are among the top 20 fruits in disease-fighting antioxidants. They can increase your good (HDL) cholesterol and lower your blood pressure, which means they may be good for your heart in more ways than one.

Ingredients
FOR THE DRESSING
¼ cup olive oil
¼ cup rice vinegar 1 tablespoon honey
¼ teaspoon pure almond extract
¼ teaspoon ground mustard Freshly ground black pepper

FOR THE SALAD
2 cups roughly chopped watercress
2 cups shredded green leaf lettuce
½ red onion, sliced very thin

½ English cucumber, chopped
1 cup sliced strawberries

Directions

TO MAKE THE DRESSING

1. In a small bowl, whisk together the olive oil and rice vinegar until emulsified.
2. Whisk in the honey, almond extract, mustard, and pepper; set aside.

TO MAKE THE SALAD

1. In a large bowl, toss together the watercress, green leaf lettuce, onion, cucumber, and strawberries.
2. Pour the dressing over the salad and toss to combine.

PER SERVING Calories: 159; Fat: 14g; Carbohydrates: 9g; Phosphorus: 34mg; Potassium: 195mg; Sodium: 14mg; Protein: 1g

CUCUMBER-DILL CABBAGE SALAD WITH LEMON DRESSING

Serves 4 / Prep time: 25 minutes, plus 1 hour to chill

The wonderfully crunchy cucumber is filled with cool, refreshing juice, making it a natural, mild diuretic. After you slice the cucumber, let it sit for 30 minutes to allow the liquid to be released from the slices. Pour off the liquid before mixing in the other ingredients. Most of the nutrition in cucumbers is found in the peel, so scrub it carefully and leave it on whenever a recipe permits. Cucumbers are a good source of vitamin A, vitamin C, and beta-carotene.

Ingredients

¼ cup heavy cream
¼ cup freshly squeezed lemon juice
2 tablespoons granulated sugar
2 tablespoons chopped fresh dill
2 tablespoons finely chopped scallion, green part only
¼ teaspoon freshly ground black pepper
1 English cucumber, sliced thin
2 cups shredded green cabbage

Directions

1. In a small bowl, stir together the cream, lemon juice, sugar, dill, scallion, and pepper until well blended.

2. In a large bowl, toss together the cucumber and cabbage.

3. Place the salad in the refrigerator and chill for 1 hour.

4. Stir before serving.

PER SERVING Calories: 99; Fat: 6g; Carbohydrates: 13g; Phosphorus: 38mg; Potassium: 200mg; Sodium: 14mg: Protein: 2g

LEAF LETTUCE AND ASPARAGUS SALAD WITH RASPBERRIES

Serves 4 / Prep time: 25 minutes

The asparagus in this recipe is raw and prepared in pretty, pale ribbons that curl around the other ingredients. Centuries ago, asparagus was considered a medicinal vegetable, especially for kidneys desease and bladder.

Asparagus acts as a natural diuretic, and it is a good source of fiber, folate, iron, and vitamins A, C, E, and K.

Ingredients

2 cups shredded green leaf lettuce
1 cup asparagus, cut into long ribbons with a peeler
1 scallion, both green and white parts, sliced
1 cup raspberries
2 tablespoons balsamic vinegar Freshly ground black pepper

Directions

1. Arrange the lettuce evenly on 4 serving plates.
2. Arrange the asparagus and scallion on top of the greens.

3. Place the raspberries on top of the salads, dividing the berries evenly.

4. Drizzle the salads with balsamic vinegar.

5. Season with pepper.

PER SERVING Calories: 36; Fat: 0g; Carbohydrates: 8g; Phosphorus: 43mg; Potassium: 200mg; Sodium: 11mg; Protein: 2g

WALDORF SALAD
Serves 4 / Prep time: 20 minutes

Waldorf salad was created in 1893 by the maître d'hôtel of the Waldorf Astoria in New York City. This original salad did not use a sour cream dressing and contained walnuts. This adaption is as spectacular as the original, and it can be topped with diced chicken if you need more protein in your diet.

Ingredients
3 cups green leaf lettuce, torn into pieces
1 cup halved grapes
3 celery stalks, chopped
1 large apple, cored, peeled, and chopped
½ cup light sour cream
2 tablespoons freshly squeezed lemon juice
1 tablespoon granulated sugar

Directions
1. Arrange the lettuce evenly on 4 plates; set aside.
2. In a small bowl, stir together the grapes, celery, and apple.
3. In another small bowl, stir together the sour cream, lemon juice, and sugar.

4. Add the sour cream mixture to the grape mixture and stir to coat.

5. Spoon the dressed grape mixture onto each plate, dividing the mixture evenly.

PER SERVING Calories: 73; Fat: 2g; Carbohydrates: 15g; Phosphorus: 29mg; Potassium: 194mg; Sodium: 30mg; Protein: 1g

ASIAN PEAR SALAD

Serves 6 / Prep time: 30 minutes, plus 1 hour to chill

Asian pears are the pale, round fruit wrapped protectively in a lacy slipcover and are found in the grocery store next to the regular pears. They look fragile but grate easily for this salad without getting mushy. These juicy, firm-textured pears add crisp sweetness to the vegetables in this slaw. You can substitute regular pears if you can't find Asian pears in your local store.

Ingredients
2 cups finely shredded green cabbage
1 cup finely shredded red cabbage
2 scallions, both green and white parts, chopped
2 celery stalks, chopped
1 Asian pear, cored and grated
½ red bell pepper, boiled and chopped
½ cup chopped cilantro
¼ cup olive oil
Juice of 1 lime
Zest of 1 lime
1 teaspoon granulated sugar

Directions

1. In a large bowl, toss together the green and red cabbage, scallions, celery, pear, red pepper, and cilantro.

2. In a small bowl, whisk together the olive oil, lime juice, lime zest, and sugar.

3. Add the dressing to the cabbage mixture and toss to combine.

4. Chill for 1 hour in the refrigerator before serving.

PER SERVING Calories: 105; Fat: 9g; Carbohydrates: 6g; Phosphorus: 17mg; Potassium: 136mg; Sodium: 48mg; Protein: 1g

COUSCOUS SALAD WITH SPICY CITRUS DRESSING

Serves 6 / Prep time: 25 minutes, plus 1 hour to chill

Couscous looks like a whole grain, but it is pasta made from semolina wheat that is steamed to a tender finish. Couscous is an ingredient found in many recipes in North Africa, and it is traditionally served topped with a meat or vegetable stew. It looks wonderfully with a variety of flavors as a main dish, side dish, or salad.

Ingredients
FOR THE DRESSING
¼ cup olive oil
3 tablespoons freshly squeezed grapefruit juice
Juice of 1 lime
Zest of 1 lime
1 tablespoon chopped fresh parsley Pinch cayenne pepper
Freshly ground black pepper

FOR THE SALAD
3 cups cooked couscous, chilled
½ red bell pepper, chopped

1 scallion, both white and green parts, chopped 1 apple, cored and chopped

Directions
TO MAKE THE DRESSING
1. In a small bowl, whisk together the olive oil, grapefruit juice, lime juice, lime zest, parsley, and cayenne pepper.
2. Season with black pepper.

TO MAKE THE SALAD
1. In a large bowl, mix together the chilled couscous, red pepper, scallion, and apple.
2. Add the dressing to the couscous mixture and toss to combine.
3. Chill in the refrigerator for at least 1 hour before serving.

Substitution tip: If you are taking a medication that prevents you from eating grapefruit, you can substitute any citrus juice, like lemon, lime, or tangerine, for grapefruit juice.

PER SERVING Calories: 187; Fat: 9g; Carbohydrates: 23g; Phosphorus: 24mg; Potassium: 108mg; Sodium: 5mg; Protein: 3g

FARFALLE CONFETTI SALAD

Serves 6 / Prep time: 30 minutes, plus 1 hour to chill

If you have a picnic or barbecue to attend, whip up this colorful dish and tote it along. The red, green, orange, and yellow vegetable flecks look pretty against the light-hued pasta and creamy dressing. Add some freshly chopped chives and a teaspoon of lemon zest as garnishes if you want an elegant finish.

Ingredients

2 cups cooked farfalle pasta

¼ cup boiled and finely chopped red bell pepper

¼ cup finely chopped cucumber

¼ cup grated carrot

2 tablespoons yellow bell pepper

½ scallion, green part only, finely chopped

½ cup Homemade Mayonnaise (here)

1 tablespoon freshly squeezed lemon juice

1 teaspoon chopped fresh parsley

½ teaspoon granulated sugar

Freshly ground black pepper

Directions

1. Mix together the pasta, red pepper, cucumber, carrot, yellow pepper, and scallion.

2. In a small bowl, whisk together the mayonnaise, lemon juice, parsley, and sugar.

3. Add the dressing to the pasta mixture and stir to combine.

4. Season with pepper.

5. Chill in the refrigerator for at least 1 hour before serving.

PER SERVING Calories: 119; Fat: 3g; Carbohydrates: 20g; Phosphorus: 51mg; Potassium: 82mg; Sodium: 16mg; Protein: 4g

TABBOULEH

Serves 6 / Prep time: 30 minutes, plus 1 hour to chill

Traditional tabbouleh features heaps of chopped herbs, usually mint, and it can be made with bulgur instead of couscous. The dressing is very simple—just a splash of olive oil and lemon juice. So use fresh juice and good-quality oil for the best results. This salad is best if it sits in the refrigerator for at least 1 hour to allow the flavors to deepen.

Ingredients
4 cups cooked white rice
½ red bell pepper, boiled and finely chopped
½ yellow bell pepper, boiled and chopped
½ zucchini, finely chopped, boiled until tender
1 cup chopped eggplant, boiled until tender
¼ cup finely chopped fresh parsley
¼ cup finely chopped fresh cilantro
2 tablespoons olive oil
Juice of 1 lemon
Zest of 1 lemon
Freshly ground black pepper

Directions

1. In a large bowl, stir together the rice, red bell pepper, yellow bell pepper, zucchini, eggplant, parsley, cilantro, olive oil, lemon juice, and lemon zest until well combined.

2. Season with pepper.

3. Chill the salad in the refrigerator for at least 1 hour before serving.

PER SERVING Calories: 177; Fat: 5g; Carbohydrates: 29g; Phosphorus: 46mg; Potassium: 189mg; Sodium: 78mg; Protein: 4g

GINGER BEEF SALAD

Serves 6 Prep time: 30 minutes, plus 1 hour to marinate; Cook time: 10 minutes

Men love this salad. It is simple, uses hot radishes and robust red onions, and sports a topping of juicy grilled beef. The beef marinade in this recipe is very spicy, so if you prefer a milder flavor, omit the chili paste. If you don't have a barbecue, the meat can be broiled for 6 minutes per side in the oven instead.

Ingredients

FOR THE BEEF
2 tablespoons olive oil
2 tablespoons freshly squeezed lime juice
1 tablespoon grated fresh ginger
2 teaspoons minced garlic
½ pound flank steak

FOR THE VINAIGRETTE
¼ cup olive oil
¼ cup rice vinegar
Juice of 1 lime
Zest of 1 lime
1 tablespoon honey
1 teaspoon chopped fresh thyme

FOR THE SALAD
4 cups torn green leaf lettuce
½ red onion, sliced thin
½ cup sliced radishes

Directions
TO MAKE THE BEEF

1. In a small bowl, stir together the olive oil, lime juice, ginger, and garlic until well blended.

2. Add the flank steak to the marinade and turn it to coat both sides of the meat.

3. Cover the bowl with plastic wrap and place in the refrigerator for 1 hour to marinate.

4. Remove the steak from the marinade and discard the marinade.

5. Preheat a barbecue to medium-high and grill the steak to medium doneness, turning once, for about 5 minutes per side, depending on the thickness of the steak.

6. Remove the steak; place on a cutting board and let the meat rest for 10 minutes.

7. Slicing the meat thinly across the grain.

TO MAKE THE VINAIGRETTE

In a small bowl, whisk together the olive oil, rice vinegar, lime juice, lime zest, honey, and thyme; set aside.

TO MAKE THE SALAD

1. Arrange the lettuce, onion, and radishes on 6 plates, dividing evenly.
2. Drizzle each salad with vinaigrette.
3. Top each salad with the sliced beef.

PER SERVING Calories: 200; Fat: 14g; Carbohydrates: 5g; Phosphorus: 84mg; Potassium: 193mg; Sodium: 29mg; Protein: 8g

KITCHEN STAPLES RECIPES

BALSAMIC VINAIGRETTE

Makes 3 cups [2 tablespoons = 1 serving] / Prep time: 5 minutes

Salads are a simple, healthy choice if you are watching your diet, so a delicious vinaigrette is a must-have. The herbs in this recipe can be switched out with your own favorites, but stick with fresh products whenever possible because dried herbs will not have as much flavor. The bright flecks of green from fresh herbs add an appealing bit of color to salad as well.

Ingredients
1½ cups extra virgin olive oil
1 cup good-quality balsamic vinegar
2 tablespoons chopped fresh parsley
2 tablespoons minced onion
1 teaspoon minced garlic

4 teaspoons chopped fresh basil Freshly ground black pepper

Directions

1. In a large bowl, whisk together the olive oil and balsamic vinegar until the ingredients emulsify, about 1 minute.
2. Whisk in the parsley, onion, garlic, and basil.
3. Season with pepper.
4. Transfer the vinaigrette to a glass jar with a lid and store at room temperature for up to 2 weeks.
5. Shake before using.

PER SERVING Calories: 129; Fat: 14g; Carbohydrates: 2g; Phosphorus: 3mg; Potassium: 16mg; Sodium: 3mg; Protein: 0g

HOMEMADE MAYONNAISE

**Makes 1 cup [1 tablespoon = 1 serving] /
Prep time: 10 minutes**

Mayonnaise is a traditional accompaniment for salads, burgers, and sandwiches. So a healthier version of the high-sodium, commercially prepared product is a handy addition to any kitchen. If you want to save a little time, whip up this recipe in a couple minutes with no whisking, using an immersion blender. Simply place your egg yolks, lemon juice, and mustard powder in a large jar that fits an immersion blender and blend for 15 seconds. Add the olive oil and blend for 15 seconds until the mayonnaise is thick and creamy.

Ingredients

2 egg yolks, at room temperature
1½ teaspoons freshly squeezed lemon juice
¼ teaspoon mustard powder
¾ cup olive oil

Directions

1. In a medium bowl, whisk together the yolks, lemon juice, and mustard for about 30 seconds or until well blended.

2. Add the olive oil in a thin, steady stream while whisking for about 3 minutes or until the oil is emulsified and the mayonnaise is thick.

3. Store the mayonnaise in the refrigerator in a sealed container for up to 1 week.

Ingredient tip: Raw eggs are used in this recipe. It should not be served to pregnant women, young children, or anyone whose immune system is compromised. The best choice for the yolks in homemade mayonnaise is washed eggs from pasture-raised chickens. Most egg food poisoning cases have come from factory-farmed chickens, and there have been no cases reported in the United States from eggs laid by pasture-raised birds.

PER SERVING Calories: 97; Fat: 11g; Carbohydrates: 0g; Phosphorus: 9mg; Potassium: 3mg; Sodium: 1mg; Protein: 0g

BALSAMIC REDUCTION

Makes ½ cup [1 tablespoon − 1 serving] / Cook time: 30 minutes

Balsamic vinegar has a rich, earthy flavor that is unmistakable and unique. This vinegar is crafted, rather than manufactured, from the pressings from grapes that are not used to make wine. The boiled-down pressings are aged under very stringent guidelines to produce balsamic vinegar. Although some balsamic vinegars are aged more than 100 years, you can use a younger, cheaper product for this reduction.

Ingredients
2 cups good-quality balsamic vinegar
1 tablespoon granulated sugar

Directions
1. Place a small saucepan over medium-high heat and whisk together the balsamic vinegar and sugar.
2. Bring the vinegar mixture to a boil.
3. Reduce the heat to low and simmer, stirring occasionally, for about 20 minutes or until the vinegar reduces.

4. Remove the vinegar reduction from the heat and allow it to cool completely.
5. Transfer the cooled reduction to a container and store at room temperature for up to 2 weeks.

Dialysis modification: Balsamic reduction is meant to add an intense burst of flavor to meats, salads, and slices of grilled bread. To reduce the amount of potassium, you can use as little as 1 teaspoon and still enjoy the delicious, rich taste.

PER SERVING Calories: 62; Fat: 0g; Carbohydrates: 12g; Phosphorus: 12mg; Potassium: 71mg; Sodium: 15mg; Protein: 0g

HERB PESTO

Makes 1½ cups [1 tablespoon = 1 serving]
Prep time: 10 minutes

Pesto can be created using a variety of base ingredients such as herbs, greens, and sun-dried tomatoes, as well as additions such as pine nuts, Parmesan cheese, and chile peppers, depending on the desired finished result. The herbs in this simple pesto are a guideline, so experiment with different choices and amounts until you get the taste you desire. Pesto is wonderful in soups and stews, as a topping for meats and poultry, or stirred into plain pasta for a simple and satisfying meal.

Ingredients

1 cup packed fresh basil leaves
½ cup packed fresh oregano leaves
½ cup packed fresh parsley leaves
2 garlic cloves
¼ cup olive oil
2 tablespoons freshly squeezed lemon juice

Directions

1. Put the basil, oregano, parsley, and garlic in a food processor and pulse for about 3 minutes or until very finely chopped.

2. Drizzle the olive oil into the pesto until a thick paste forms, scraping down the sides at least once.

3. Add the lemon juice and pulse until well blended.

4. Store the pesto in a sealed container in the refrigerator for up to 1 week.

PER SERVING Calories: 22; Fat: 2g; Carbohydrates: 0g; Phosphorus: 2mg; Potassium: 15mg; Sodium: 1mg; Protein: 0g

ALFREDO SAUCE

Serves 8 [¼ cup = 1 serving] Prep time: 10 minutes; Cook time: 10 minutes

Creamy pasta sauces are typically a sauce to be eaten on special occasions. This recipe tastes just as cheesy and creamy but without the hefty amounts of fat, calories, phosphorus, or sodium, so you can enjoy the sauce more often with family and friends. Wipe the bowl out with a chunk of crusty bread to soak up every last drop

Ingredients
2 tablespoons unsalted butter
1½ tablespoons all-purpose flour
1 teaspoon minced garlic
1 cup plain unsweetened rice milk
¾ cup plain cream cheese
2 tablespoons Parmesan cheese
¼ teaspoon ground nutmeg
Freshly ground black pepper, for seasoning

Directions

1. In a medium saucepan over medium heat, melt the butter.

2. Whisk in the flour and garlic to form a paste, and continue whisking for 2 minutes to cook the flour.

3. Whisk in the rice milk and continue whisking for about 4 minutes or until the mixture is almost boiling and thick.

4. Whisk in the cream cheese, Parmesan cheese, and nutmeg for about 1 minute or until the sauce is smooth.

5. Remove the sauce from the heat and season with pepper.

6. Serve immediately over pasta.

PER SERVING Calories: 98; Fat: 7g; Carbohydrates: 6g; Phosphorus: 66mg; Potassium: 70mg; Sodium: 141mg; Protein: 3g

APPLE-CRANBERRY CHUTNEY

Makes 1 cup [1 tablespoon − 1 serving]
Prep time: 10 minutes; Cook time: 30 minutes

Chutneys sound old-fashioned and sweet, but most chutneys have complex flavors that range from mouth-scorching spicy to lip-puckering tart with only a hint of sweetness. This chutney is a milder variation that perfectly balances sweet and tart. You should keep a jar handy for chicken and pork recipes, as well as for a tasty snack on top of crackers.

Ingredients

1 large apple, peeled, cored, and sliced thin
½ cup granulated sugar
½ cup fresh cranberries
½ red onion, finely chopped
¼ cup apple juice
¼ cup apple cider vinegar
Freshly ground black pepper, for seasoning

Directions

1. In a medium saucepan over medium heat, stir together the apple, sugar, cranberries, onion, apple juice, and vinegar.

2. Bring the mixture to a boil, and then reduce the heat to low and cook, stirring frequently, for 25 to 30 minutes or until the cranberries are very tender.

3. Season with pepper.

4. Remove the chutney from the heat and chill in the refrigerator for about 3 hours or until completely cool.

5. Store the chutney in a sealed container in the refrigerator for up to 1 week.

PER SERVING Calories: 36; Fat: 0g; Carbohydrates: 9g; Phosphorus: 3mg; Potassium: 25mg; Sodium: 1mg; Protein: 0g

COOKED FOUR-PEPPER SALSA

Makes 4 cups [½ cup = 1 serving] Prep time: 15 minutes; Cook time: 1 hour, 15 minutes

Red bell peppers are a popular choice if you are following a renal diet because they are low in potassium. This pretty-hued vegetable is also a nutritional powerhouse because it is an excellent source of vitamins A and C (both antioxidants), vitamin E, vitamin B6, folate, and fiber. Red bell peppers also contain the antioxidants lycopene, and beta-cryptoxanthin, which offer protection against heart disease and lung cancer.

Ingredients

1 pound red bell peppers, boiled and chopped
2 small sweet banana peppers, chopped
1 small sweet onion, chopped
1 jalapeño pepper, finely chopped
1 green bell pepper, chopped
½ cup apple cider vinegar
2 teaspoons minced garlic
1 tablespoon granulated sugar
3 tablespoons chopped fresh cilantro

Directions

1. In a large saucepan, mix together the red bell peppers, banana peppers, onion, jalapeño pepper, green bell pepper, apple cider vinegar, garlic, and sugar over medium heat.

2. Bring the mixture to a boil, stirring frequently.

3. Reduce the heat to low and simmer for about 1 hour, stirring frequently.

4. Stir in the cilantro and simmer, stirring occasionally, for 15 minutes.

5. Remove the salsa from the heat and allow it to cool 15 to 20 minutes.

6. Transfer the salsa to a container and chill in the refrigerator until you are ready to use it, up to 1 week.

7. Serve cold with baked tortilla chips.

PER SERVING Calories: 40; Fat: 0g; Carbohydrates: 8g; Phosphorus: 24mg; Potassium: 191mg; Sodium: 4mg; Protein: 1g

EASY CHICKEN STOCK

Makes 8 to 10 cups [1 cup = 1 serving]
Prep time: 15 minutes; Cook time: 7 to 8 hours

Making chicken stock is an art that requires a large stockpot and patience. The ingredients for this recipe are very flexible, so omit or add whatever you want as long as the carcass, water, and vinegar remain. The vinegar draws out important nutrients from the chicken bones that enhance the health benefits of making your own stock. If you use a raw carcass, roast the bones in the oven for a few hours to enhance the flavor before adding the carcass to your stockpot.

Ingredients

1 roasted chicken carcass, skin removed
Water
1 tablespoon apple cider vinegar
4 celery stalks, chopped into 2-inch pieces
2 sweet onions, peeled and quartered
2 carrots, cut into 2-inch chunks
2 garlic cloves, crushed
2 bay leaves
5 fresh thyme sprigs
5 fresh parsley stems

½ teaspoon black peppercorns

Directions

1. Put the chicken carcass in a large 4-to 6-quart stockpot, cutting it into smaller pieces to make it fit, if needed.

2. Cover the carcass with water until the liquid covers the carcass by about 1 inch, and add the apple cider vinegar.

3. Place the stockpot over medium heat until the liquid simmers and then reduce the heat to low so that it simmers very gently.

4. Simmer the carcass for 5 to 6 hours, adding more water if the top of the carcass gets exposed.

5. Skim off any accumulated foam on the stock.

6. Add the celery, onion, carrots, garlic, bay leaves, thyme, parsley, and peppercorns to the stockpot.

7. Simmer for 2 hours, adding more water if required to keep the ingredients covered.

8. Strain the stock through a fine-mesh strainer and discard the solids.

9. Let the stock cool, and store in the refrigerator for up to 1 week or in the freezer for up to 6 months.

Dialysis modification: When the stock is finished, add water to increase the volume and reduce the amount of potassium. As many as 3 or 4 cups of water will not dilute the chicken taste too much, but make sure to taste as you add water to reach an acceptable flavor.

PER SERVING Calories: 38; Fat: 1g; Carbohydrates: 3g; Phosphorus: 72mg; Potassium: 197mg; Sodium: 72mg; Protein: 5g

CINNAMON APPLESAUCE

Makes 3 cups [½ cup = 1 serving] Prep time: 10 minutes; Cook time: 30 minutes

Applesauce is a comfort food in a healthy package. The sweet, slightly tart, spiced goodness of this dish is perfect for a nutrition-packed snack, as breakfast, or even spooned over a simple grilled pork chop. Apples are full of fiber and rich in antioxidants. This recipe is even sweeter if you need to use up apples that are a wee bit past their prime.

Ingredients

8 apples, peeled, cored, and sliced thin
½ cup water
1 teaspoon ground cinnamon
¼ teaspoon ground nutmeg Pinch ground allspice

Directions

1. Put the apples, water, cinnamon, nutmeg, and allspice in a medium saucepan over medium heat.
2. Heat the apple mixture, stirring frequently, for 25 to 30 minutes, or until the apples soften.

3. Remove the saucepan from the heat and use a potato masher to mash the apples to the desired texture.

4. Let the applesauce cool.

5. Store in the refrigerator for up to 1 week.

PER SERVING Calories: 106; Fat: 0g; Carbohydrates: 28g; Phosphorus: 24mg; Potassium: 196mg; Sodium: 0g; Protein: 1g

LEMON CURD

Makes 1½ cups [2 tablespoons = 1 serving] Prep time: 15 minutes; Cook time: 10 minutes

Lemon is one of the most popular taste profiles in the world, across many different cultures. This velvety curd has an intense lemon flavor accented by a touch of sweetness and rich butter. You can spread lemon curd on toast, fold it into whipped topping for a light dessert, or use it to top a bowl of fresh berries. Lemons are an excellent source of limonene, which has been shown to have antioxidant properties.

Lemons also are an excellent source of vitamin C and folate.

Ingredients

6 large egg yolks
¾ cup granulated sugar
Zest of 4 lemons
Juice of 4 lemons
½ cup unsalted butter, cut into 1-inch pieces

Directions

1. Pour about 2 inches of water into a small saucepan and place over medium- high heat until the water simmers.

2. Reduce the heat to low so the water gently simmers, and place a medium stainless-steel bowl over the saucepan.

3. In the bowl, whisk together the egg yolks, sugar, lemon zest, and lemon juice for 8 to 10 minutes or until the mixture forms thick ribbons when you lift up the whisk.

4. Remove the bowl from the saucepan and whisk in the butter pieces, one at a time, until each is fully incorporated.

5. Pour the lemon curd through a fine-mesh strainer into another medium bowl. Use the back of a spoon to press through extra curd and squeeze out the zest.

6. Discard the zest in the strainer, and cover the lemon curd with plastic wrap that is pressed right onto the surface of the curd.

7. Chill in the refrigerator for about 3 hours or until set.

8. Store in the refrigerator in a sealed container for up to 1 week.

PER SERVING Calories: 148; Fat: 10g; Carbohydrates: 14g; Phosphorus: 37mg; Potassium: 32mg; Sodium: 5g; Protein: 1g

TRADITIONAL BEEF STOCK

Makes 8 cups [1 cup = 1 serving] Prep time: 15 minutes; Cook time: 13 hours

Most grocery stores have bones in their meat sections because bone broth and a back-to-basics attitude about diet has created a demand for this ingredient. You can also visit a butcher or a farmers' market to find good quality beef bones.

Ingredients

2 pounds beef bones (beef marrow, knuckle bones, or ribs)
1 celery stalk, chopped into 2-inch pieces
1 carrot, peeled and roughly chopped
½ sweet onion, peeled and quartered
3 garlic cloves, crushed
1 teaspoon black peppercorns
3 sprigs thyme
2 bay leaves Water

Directions

1. Preheat the oven to 350°F.
2. Place the bones in a deep baking pan and roast them in the oven for 30 minutes, turning once.

3. Transfer the roasted bones to a large stockpot and add the celery, carrots, onion, garlic, peppercorns, thyme, bay leaves, and enough water to cover the bones by about 3 inches.

4. Reduce the heat to low and simmer the stock for at least 12 hours. Check the broth every hour for the first 4 hours to skim off any foam or impurities from the top.

5. Remove the pot from the heat and cool for 30 minutes.

6. Remove the large bones with tongs, and then strain the stock through a fine- mesh strainer and discard the solid bits in the strainer.

7. Pour the stock into jars or containers and allow it to cool completely.

8. Store the beef stock in sealed containers or jars in the refrigerator for up to 6 days, or in the freezer for up to 3 months.

PER SERVING Calories: 121; Fat: 5g; Carbohydrates: 2g; Phosphorus: 21mg; Potassium: 79mg; Sodium: 87mg; Protein: 4g

SPICE BLENDS AND SEASONINGS

FAJITA RUB

Makes ¼ cup [½ teaspoon = 1 serving] / Prep time: 5 minutes

Tex-Mex food is so popular in fine-dining restaurants across North America. Fajitas are one of the classic offerings in establishments featuring this cuisine. This combination of spices originated with Mexican workers in Texas in the 1930s, when they were given less-desirable cuts of beef such as flank or skirt steaks when steers were slaughtered. In Spanish, the word for girdle is faja, which is the root of fajita.

Ingredients
1½ teaspoons chili powder
1 teaspoon garlic powder
1 teaspoon roasted cumin seed
1 teaspoon dried oregano
½ teaspoon ground coriander
¼ teaspoon red pepper flakes

Directions

1. Put the chili powder, garlic powder, cumin seed, oregano, coriander, and red pepper flakes in a blender, and pulse until the ingredients are ground and well combined.

2. Transfer the spice mixture to a small container with a lid.

3. Store in a cool, dry place for up to 6 months.

PER SERVING Calories: 1; Fat: 0g; Carbohydrates: 0g; Phosphorus: 2mg; Potassium: 7mg; Sodium: 7mg; Protein: 0g

DRIED HERB RUB

**Makes ⅓ cup [½ teaspoon = 1 serving] /
Prep time: 5 minutes**

The combination of herbs in this recipe can
be changed according to your palate and
depending on what you have in your pantry.
Chicken, pork, and firm white fish are
enhanced with a generous sprinkling of this
mixture before grilling or baking. You can
easily double the recipe if you find yourself
using a lot of the rub.

Ingredients
1 tablespoon dried thyme
1 tablespoon dried oregano
1 tablespoon dried parsley
2 teaspoons dried basil
2 teaspoons ground coriander
2 teaspoons onion powder
1 teaspoon ground cumin
1 teaspoon garlic powder
1 teaspoon paprika
½ teaspoon cayenne pepper

Directions

1. Put the thyme, oregano, parsley, basil, coriander, onion powder, cumin, garlic powder, paprika, and cayenne pepper in a blender, and press until the ingredients are ground and well combined.

2. Transfer the rub to a small container with a lid.

3. Store in a cool, dry place for up to 6 months.

PER SERVING Calories: 3; Fat: 0g; Carbohydrates: 1g; Phosphorus: 3mg; Potassium: 16mg; Sodium: 1mg; Protein: 0g

MEDITERRANEAN SEASONING

**Makes ⅓ cup [½ teaspoon = 1 serving] /
Prep time: 5 minutes**

This Mediterranean-inspired seasoning may conjure up images of sun-drenched patios, clear waters, and flavorful fresh food. Oregano is a popular herb in Greek cuisine and can be found growing in almost every kitchen garden in that country. Do not omit oregano from the seasoning mix if you want an authentic taste.

Ingredients
2 tablespoons dried oregano
1 tablespoon dried thyme
2 teaspoons dried rosemary, chopped finely or crushed
2 teaspoons dried basil
1 teaspoon dried marjoram
1 teaspoon dried parsley flakes

Directions
1. In a small bowl, mix together the oregano, thyme, rosemary, basil, marjoram, and parsley until well combined.

2. Transfer the seasoning mixture to a small container with a lid.

3. Store in a cool, dry place for up to 6 months.

PER SERVING Calories: 1; Fat: 0g; Carbohydrates: 0g; Phosphorus: 1mg; Potassium: 6mg; Sodium: 0mg; Protein: 0g

HOT CURRY POWDER

Makes 1¼ cups [1 tablespoon = 1 serving]
Prep time: 5 minutes

The curry powder found in jars at the supermarket is a complex mix of many spices—not a single ingredient. A traditional South Asian curry contains turmeric, cumin, and coriander, with other spices thrown in depending on the region.

Ingredients
¼ cup ground cumin
¼ cup ground coriander
3 tablespoons turmeric
2 tablespoons sweet paprika
2 tablespoons of ground mustard

1 tablespoon of fennel powder
½ teaspoon green chili powder
2 teaspoons ground cardamom 1 teaspoon ground cinnamon
½ teaspoon ground cloves

Directions

1. Put the cumin, coriander, turmeric, paprika, mustard, fennel powder, green chili powder, cardamom, cinnamon, and cloves into a blender, and press until the ingredients are ground and well combined.

2. Transfer the curry powder to a small container with a lid.

3. Store in a cool, dry place for up to 6 months.

Dialysis modification: Omit the sweet paprika to reduce the amount of potassium. It will change the color of the curry powder, but the other spices have a strong enough flavor to make up for the omission.

PER SERVING Calories: 19; Fat: 1g; Carbohydrates: 3g; Phosphorus: 24mg; Potassium: 93mg; Sodium: 5mg; Protein: 1g

CAJUN SEASONING

Makes 1¼ cups [1 teaspoon = 1 serving] / Prep time: 5 minutes

Cajun cooking is native to Louisiana in the United States, but the original Cajuns were French people from Nova Scotia (Acadia) who were forced out of Canada by the British in 1755. A large group settled in south Louisiana and was eventually joined by more Cajuns looking for a safe haven. Cajun food is spicy, garlicky, and often features grilled meats or wild game.

Ingredients

½ cup sweet paprika
¼ cup garlic powder
3 tablespoons onion powder
3 tablespoons freshly ground black pepper
2 tablespoons dried oregano
1 tablespoon cayenne pepper
1 tablespoon dried thyme

Directions

1. Put the paprika, garlic powder, onion powder, black pepper, oregano, cayenne pepper, and thyme in a blender, and pulse until the ingredients are ground and well combined.

2. Transfer the seasoning mixture to a small container with a lid.

3. Store in a cool, dry place for up to 6 months.

PER SERVING Calories: 7; Fat: 0g; Carbohydrates: 2g; Phosphorus: 8mg; Potassium: 40mg; Sodium: 1mg; Protein: 0g

APPLE PIE SPICE

**Makes ⅓ cup [1 teaspoon − 1 serving] /
Prep time: 5 minutes**

If you use pumpkin pie spice, this blend will taste and smell familiar. Pumpkins are not recommended on a renal diet, but apple pie can fill in. This spice mix can also be added to ½ cup of granulated sugar to create a delicious topping for hot buttered toast when you need a treat.

Ingredients

¼ cup ground cinnamon
2 teaspoons ground nutmeg
2 teaspoons ground ginger
1 teaspoon allspice
½ teaspoon ground cloves

Directions

1. In a small bowl, mix together the cinnamon, nutmeg, ginger, allspice, and cloves until the ingredients are well combined.
2. Transfer the spice mixture to a small container with a lid.
3. Store in a cool, dry place for up to 6 months.

PER SERVING Calories: 6; Fat: 0g; Carbohydrates: 1g; Phosphorus: 2mg; Potassium: 12mg; Sodium: 1mg; Protein: 0g

RAS EL HANOUT

Makes ½ cup [1 teaspoon = 1 serving] / Prep time: 5 minutes

Spices are a way of life in many North African regions, and the intoxicating scent of spice markets lingers in city streets. Many variations of ras el hanout spice mix exist. Some are tightly held secrets of families and restaurants in North Africa. Some variations include up to 100 different spices in the blend. This recipe is a simple version of the traditional mixture.

Ingredients
2 teaspoons ground nutmeg
2 teaspoons ground coriander
2 teaspoons ground cumin
2 teaspoons turmeric
2 teaspoons cinnamon
1 teaspoon cardamom

1 teaspoon sweet paprika
1 teaspoon ground mace
1 teaspoon freshly ground black pepper
1 teaspoon cayenne pepper
½ teaspoon ground allspice
½ teaspoon ground cloves

Directions

1. In a small bowl, mix together the nutmeg, coriander, cumin, turmeric, cinnamon, cardamom, paprika, mace, black pepper, cayenne pepper, allspice, and cloves until the ingredients are well combined.
2. Transfer the seasoning mixture to a small container with a lid.
3. Store in a cool, dry place for up to 6 months.

PER SERVING Calories: 5; Fat: 0g; Carbohydrates: 1g; Phosphorus: 3mg; Potassium: 17mg; Sodium: 1mg; Protein: 0g

POULTRY SEASONING

Makes ½ cup [1 teaspoon = 1 serving] / Prep time: 5 minutes

Commercially prepared poultry seasonings are often very high in sodium because salt is thought to draw the juices out of the bird to produce a crackly, golden skin. Salt does draw the juices out of chicken and turkey, but you do not need it to create a lovely meal. Celery seed adds a salty flavor to this blend without the sodium.

Ingredients
2 tablespoons ground thyme
2 tablespoons ground marjoram
1 tablespoon ground sage
1 tablespoon ground celery seed
1 teaspoon ground rosemary
1 teaspoon freshly ground black pepper

Directions
1. In a small bowl, mix together the thyme, marjoram, sage, celery seed, rosemary, and pepper until the ingredients are well combined.

2. Transfer the seasoning mixture to a small container with a lid.
3. Store in a cool, dry place for up to 6 months.

PER SERVING Calories: 3; Fat: 0g; Carbohydrates: 0g; Phosphorus: 3mg; Potassium: 10mg; Sodium: 1mg; Protein: 0g

BERBERE SPICE MIX

Makes ½ cup [1 teaspoon = 1 serving] Prep time: 5 minutes; Cook time: 5 minutes

This spice mix takes a little more work than just mixing ingredients in a bowl, but the result is worth all the effort. Berbere has its roots in Ethiopia, where its fiery taste is familiar even to children. Do not exclude the fenugreek seeds and dried chiles if you want to try an authentic-flavored blend.

Ingredients
1 tablespoon coriander seeds
1 teaspoon cumin seeds
1 teaspoon fenugreek seeds

¼ teaspoon black peppercorns
¼ teaspoon whole allspice berries
4 whole cloves
4 dried chiles, stemmed and seeded
¼ cup dried onion flakes
2 tablespoons ground cardamom
1 tablespoon sweet paprika
1 teaspoon ground ginger
½ teaspoon ground nutmeg
½ teaspoon ground cinnamon

Directions

1. In a small skillet over medium heat, add the coriander, cumin, fenugreek, peppercorns, allspice, and cloves.

2. Lightly toast the spices, swirling the skillet constantly, for about 4 minutes or until the spices are fragrant.

3. Remove the skillet from the heat and let the spices cool for about 10 minutes.

4. Transfer the toasted spices to a blender with the chiles and onion, and grind until the mixture is finely ground.

5. Transfer the ground spice mixture to a small bowl and stir together the cardamom, paprika, ginger, nutmeg, and cinnamon until thoroughly combined.

6. Store the spice mixture in a small container with a lid for up to 6 months.

PER SERVING Calories: 8; Fat: 0g; Carbohydrates. 2g; Phosphorus: 7mg; Potassium: 37mg; Sodium: 14mg; Protein: 0g

CREOLE SEASONING MIX

Makes ¼ cup [1 teaspoon = 1 serving] / Prep time: 5 minutes

Creole food is the urban equivalent of the more rural Cajun cuisine in Louisiana. Traditional Creole food uses tomatoes, which are not recommended on a renal diet, but you can still enjoy using this seasoning mix in recipes despite the tomato omission. Creole cuisine uses many high-quality ingredients made popular in upscale kitchens in New Orleans.

Ingredients

1 tablespoon sweet paprika
1 tablespoon garlic powder
2 teaspoons onion powder
2 teaspoons dried oregano
1 teaspoon cayenne pepper

1 teaspoon ground thyme
1 teaspoon freshly ground black pepper

Directions

1. In a small bowl, mix together the paprika, garlic powder, onion powder, oregano, cayenne pepper, thyme, and black pepper until the ingredients are well combined.

2. Transfer the seasoning mixture to a small container with a lid.

3. Store in a cool, dry place for up to 6 months.

PER SERVING Calories: 7; Fat: 0g; Carbohydrates: 2g; Phosphorus: 8mg; Potassium: 35mg; Sodium: 1mg; Protein: 0g

ADOBO SEASONING MIX

**Makes 1¼ cups [1 teaspoon = 1 serving] /
Prep time: 5 minutes**

This mix varies depending on the region and it is often used for meats and poultry, and as a marinade base for peppers or other vegetables. Dried citrus zest can be added to the mix for a Puerto Rican flair, or you can mix this blend with lemon juice or vinegar to create a wet rub for fish or pork.

Ingredients

4 tablespoons garlic powder
4 tablespoons onion powder
4 tablespoons ground cumin
3 tablespoons dried oregano
3 tablespoons freshly ground black pepper
2 tablespoons sweet paprika
2 tablespoons ground chili powder
1 tablespoon ground turmeric
1 tablespoon ground coriander

Directions

1. In a small bowl, mix together the garlic powder, onion powder, cumin, oregano, black pepper, paprika, chili powder, turmeric, and coriander until the ingredients are well combined.

2. Transfer the seasoning mixture to a small container with a lid and store in a cool, dry place for up to 6 months.

PER SERVING Calories: 8; Fat: 0g; Carbohydrates: 2g; Phosphorus: 9mg; Potassium: 38mg; Sodium: 12mg; Protein: 0g

HERBES DE PROVENCE

**Makes 1 cup [1 teaspoon = 1 serving] /
Prep time: 5 minutes**

The banks of purple lavender stretching for miles in the French countryside are a breathtaking reminder that this fragrant flower is also delicious in food. You do not have to include lavender in this mix, but because of its unique flavor and because you can purchase easily online, why leave it out? Make sure you purchase organic, culinary-grade lavender to avoid pesticide or chemical contamination.

Ingredients
½ cup dried thyme
3 tablespoons dried marjoram
3 tablespoons dried savory
2 tablespoons dried rosemary
2 teaspoons dried lavender flowers
1 teaspoon ground fennel

Directions

1. Put the thyme, marjoram, savory, rosemary, lavender, and fennel in a blender and pulse a few times to combine.

2. Transfer the herb mixture to a small container with a lid.

3. Store in a cool, dry place for up to 6 months.

PER SERVING Calories: 3; Fat: 0g; Carbohydrates: 1g; Phosphorus: 2mg; Potassium: 9mg; Sodium: 0mg; Protein: 0g

LAMB AND PORK SEASONING

**Makes ½ cup [1 teaspoon = 1 serving] /
Prep time: 5 minutes**

Meats often need more assertive spicing than delicate fish or poultry, so seasoning with celery seed, onion, garlic, and lots of black pepper creates just the right taste. Bay leaves are often used whole in stews, soups, and sauces, but they can also be found ground in the spice section of most supermarkets.

Ingredients
¼ cup celery seed
2 tablespoons dried oregano
2 tablespoons onion powder
1 tablespoon dried thyme
1½ teaspoons garlic powder
1 teaspoon crushed bay leaf
1 teaspoon freshly ground black pepper
1 teaspoon ground allspice

Directions
1. Put the celery seed, oregano, onion powder, thyme, garlic powder, bay leaf, pepper, and all spices in a blender and pulse a few times to combine.

2. Transfer the herb mixture to a small container with a lid.
3. Store in a cool, dry place for up to 6 months.

PER SERVING Calories: 8; Fat: 0g; Carbohydrates: 1g; Phosphorus: 9mg; Potassium: 29mg; Sodium: 2mg; Protein: 0g

ASIAN SEASONING

**Makes ½ cup [1 teaspoon = 1 serving] /
Prep time: 5 minutes**

Toasty-flavored sesame and exotic licorice-flavored anise combine with a mix of fragrant spices to create a seasoning blend that might become your new favorite. Seeds are not usually allowed if you are following a renal diet, but the quantity in this mix is tiny when divided into teaspoon-sized servings. You can omit the sesame seeds, but the loss in flavor will be significant.

Ingredients

2 tablespoons sesame seeds
2 tablespoons onion powder
2 tablespoons crushed star anise pods
2 tablespoons ground ginger
1 teaspoon ground allspice
½ teaspoon cardamom
½ teaspoon ground cloves

Directions

1. In a small bowl, mix together the sesame seeds, onion powder, star anise, ginger, allspice, cardamom, and cloves until well combined.

2. Transfer the spice mixture to a small container with a lid.

3. Store in a cool, dry place for up to 6 months.

PER SERVING Calories: 10; Fat: 0g; Carbohydrates: 1g; Phosphorus: 11mg; Potassium: 24mg; Sodium: 5mg; Protein: 0g

ONION SEASONING BLEND

Makes ½ cup [1 teaspoon = 1 serving] / Prep time: 5 minutes

Onion powder has an intense flavor without any of the bite that can be found in fresh onions. This seasoning blend has an unexpected sweet undertone, which is perfect for pork or sprinkling on roasted vegetables. You can also enjoy the taste of onions without the crying that can happen when cutting fresh alliums.

Ingredients
2 tablespoons onion powder
1 tablespoon dry mustard
2 teaspoons sweet paprika

2 teaspoons garlic powder
1 teaspoon dried thyme
½ teaspoon celery seeds
½ teaspoon freshly ground black pepper

Directions

1. In a small bowl, mix together the onion powder, mustard, paprika, garlic powder, thyme, celery seeds, and pepper until well combined.
2. Transfer the spice mixture to a small container with a lid.
3. Store in a cool, dry place for up to 6 months.

PER SERVING Calories: 5; Fat: 0g; Carbohydrates: 1g; Phosphorus: 6mg; Potassium: 17mg; Sodium: 1mg; Protein: 1g

COFFEE DRY RUB

**Makes ¼ cup [1 teaspoon = 1 serving] /
Prep time: 5 minutes**

Coffee is typically something you enjoy in a mug in the morning. However, coffee adds a complexity to any flavoring mix and enhances the natural taste of beef. If you have a coffee grinder, grind your coffee right before mixing this rub together so the taste is intense.

Ingredients
1 tablespoon ground coffee
2 teaspoons ground cumin
2 teaspoons sweet paprika
2 teaspoons chili powder
1 teaspoon brown sugar
¼ teaspoon freshly ground black pepper

Directions
1. In a small bowl, mix together the coffee, cumin, paprika, chili powder, brown sugar, and pepper until well combined.
2. Transfer the rub to a small container with a lid.
3. Store in a cool, dry place for up to 6 months.

PER SERVING Calories: 5; Fat: 0g; Carbohydrates: 1g; Phosphorus: 5mg; Potassium: 32mg; Sodium: 18mg; Protein: 0g

VEGETARIANS ENTREES

EGG WHITE FRITTATA WITH PENNE

Serves 4 Prep time: 15 minutes Cook time: 30 minutes

A frittata is one of the easiest ways to prepare eggs, and the results look like you've spent hours in the kitchen. Even if you make frittatas all the time, adding pasta may be a new twist. Pasta creates a heartier dish that is perfect for lunch on a busy weekend or cut up into squares for a road trip.

Ingredients
6 egg whites
¼ cup rice milk
1 tablespoon chopped fresh parsley
1 teaspoon chopped fresh thyme
1 teaspoon chopped fresh chives
Freshly ground black pepper
2 teaspoons olive oil
¼ small sweet onion, chopped

1 teaspoon minced garlic
½ cup boiled and chopped red bell pepper
2 cups cooked penne

Directions

1. Preheat the oven to 350°F.
2. In a large bowl, whisk together the egg whites, rice milk, parsley, thyme, chives, and pepper.
3. In a large ovenproof skillet over medium heat, heat the olive oil.
4. Sauté the onion, garlic, and red pepper for about 4 minutes or until they are softened.
5. Using a spatula, add the cooked penne to the skillet to evenly distribute the pasta.
6. Pour the egg mixture over the pasta and shake the pan to coat the pasta.
7. Leave the skillet on the heat for 1 minute to set the bottom of the frittata and then transfer the skillet to the oven.
8. Bake the frittata for about 25 minutes or until it is set and golden brown.
9. Remove from the oven and serve immediately.

PER SERVING Calories: 170; Fat: 3g; Carbohydrates: 25g; Phosphorus: 62mg; Potassium: 144mg; Sodium: 90mg; Protein: 10g

VEGETABLE FRIED RICE

Serves 6 Prep time: 20 minutes Cook time: 20 minutes

If you find fried rice in restaurants is too greasy and salty, this fresh, flavorful dish will be a satisfying treat. For a more substantial dish, add two beaten eggs scrambled right in the pan at the end. Push the rice and vegetables aside, creating an empty spot in the skillet, and scramble the eggs before stirring them back into the rice mixture. This will add about 30 mg of phosphorus and 20 mg of potassium to each serving.

Ingredients

1 tablespoon olive oil

½ sweet onion, chopped
1 tablespoon grated fresh ginger
 2 teaspoons minced garlic
1 cup sliced carrots
½ cup chopped eggplant
½ cup peas
½ cup green beans, cut into 1-inch pieces
2 tablespoons chopped fresh cilantro
3 cups cooked rice

Directions

1. In a large skillet over medium-high heat, heat the olive oil.

2. Sauté the onion, ginger, and garlic for about 3 minutes or until softened.

3. Stir in the carrot, eggplant, peas, and green beans and sauté for 3 minutes more.

4. Add the cilantro and rice.

5. Sauté, stirring constantly, for about 10 minutes or until the rice is heated through.

6. Serve immediately.

PER SERVING Calories: 189; Fat: 7g; Carbohydrates: 28g; Phosphorus: 89mg; Potassium: 172mg; Sodium: 13mg; Protein: 6g

BULGUR-STUFFED SPAGHETTI SQUASH

Serves 4 Prep time: 20 minutes Cook time: 50 minutes

Golden squash makes a convenient and pretty container to hold vegetables, grains, spices, and fruit. The most important part of creating this meal is to make sure you don't pierce the skin while scooping out the roasted flesh. A hole in the squash shell will allow the juices and filling to escape.

Ingredients
FOR THE SQUASH
2 small spaghetti squash, halved
1 teaspoon olive oil
Freshly ground black pepper

FOR THE FILLING
1 teaspoon olive oil
½ small sweet onion, finely diced
1 teaspoon minced garlic
½ cup chopped carrot
½ cup cranberries
1 teaspoon chopped fresh thyme
½ teaspoon ground cumin
½ teaspoon ground coriander

Juice of ½ lemon

1 cup cooked bulgur

Directions

TO MAKE THE SQUASH

1. Preheat the oven to 350°F.

2. Line a baking sheet with parchment paper.

3. Lightly oil the cut sides of the squash, season with pepper, and place them cut-side down on the baking sheet.

4. Bake for 25 to 30 minutes or until tender. Remove the squash from the oven and flip the squash halves over.

5. Scoop out the flesh from each half, leaving about ½ inch around the edges and keeping the skin intact.

6. Place 2 cups of squash flesh in a large bowl and reserve the rest for another recipe.

TO MAKE THE FILLING

1. In a medium skillet over medium heat, heat the olive oil.

2. Sauté the onion, garlic, carrot, and cranberries for 5 to 6 minutes or until softened.

3. Add the sautéed vegetables to the squash in the bowl.

4. Add the thyme, cumin, and coriander, stirring to combine.

5. Stir in the lemon juice and cooked bulgur until well mixed.

6. Spoon the filling evenly into the squash halves.

7. Bake in the oven for about 15 minutes or until heated through.

8. Serve warm.

PER SERVING Calories: 111; Fat: 2g; Carbohydrates: 17g; Phosphorus: 38mg; Potassium: 182mg; Sodium: 22mg; Protein: 3g

RED PEPPER STRATA

Serves 8 Prep time: 20 minutes, plus 2 hours soaking time; Cook time: 1 hour, 5 minutes

Centuries ago, savory bread pudding was a tasty way to use up stale bread, leftovers, and eggs when serving large groups of people. This dish can be doubled easily, other vegetables can be added, and it can be prepared the night before for convenience. If you want enhanced flavor, use a homemade, herb- infused vinegar.

Ingredients
Butter, for greasing the baking dish
8 slices fresh white bread, cut into cubes
1 tablespoon unsalted butter
½ sweet onion, chopped
1 teaspoon minced garlic
1 red bell pepper, boiled and chopped
6 eggs
¼ cup tarragon vinegar
1 cup rice milk
1 teaspoon Tabasco sauce
½ teaspoon freshly ground black pepper

1 ounce Parmesan cheese, grated

Directions
1. Preheat the oven to 250°F.
2. Lightly grease a 9-by-9-inch baking dish with butter; set aside.
3. Line a baking sheet with parchment paper and scatter the bread cubes on the sheet.
4. Bake the bread cubes for about 10 minutes or until they are crisp.
5. Remove the bread cubes from the oven; set aside.
6. In a medium skillet over medium-high heat, melt the butter.
7. Sauté the onion and garlic for about 3 minutes or until softened.
8. Add the red pepper and sauté an additional 2 minutes.
9. Spread half of the bread cubes in a layer in the baking dish and top with half of the sautéed vegetables.
10. Repeat with the remaining half of the bread cubes and vegetables.
11. In a medium bowl, whisk together the eggs, vinegar, rice milk, hot sauce, and pepper.
12. Pour the egg mixture evenly into the baking dish.

13. Cover the dish and place in the fridge to soak for at least 2 hours or overnight.

14. Let the strata come to room temperature.

15. Preheat the oven to 325°F.

16. Remove the plastic wrap and bake for about 45 minutes or until golden.

17. Sprinkle the top of the strata with cheese and bake an additional 5 minutes.

18. Serve hot.

PER SERVING Calories: 150; Fat: 6g; Carbohydrates: 10g; Phosphorus: 120mg; Potassium: 89mg; Sodium: 168mg; Protein: 7g

COUSCOUS BURGERS

**Serves 4 Prep time: 20 minutes, plus 1
hour chilling time; Cook time: 10 minutes**

Veggie burgers have a bad reputation
because they are often tasteless and dry or
have a strange texture. Couscous is a
delightfully tender base, especially when
infused with citrus and herbs. You can make
a double batch and freeze the uncooked
patties for up to 3 months for a quick and
convenient meal. Serve them alone or on a
bun with your favorite toppings.

ingredients
½ cup canned chickpeas, rinsed and drained
2 tablespoons chopped fresh cilantro
2 tablespoons chopped fresh parsley
1 tablespoon freshly squeezed lemon juice
2 teaspoons lemon zest
1 teaspoon minced garlic
2½ cups cooked couscous
2 eggs, lightly beaten
2 tablespoons olive oil

Directions

1. Put the chickpeas, cilantro, parsley, lemon juice, lemon zest, and garlic in a food processor and pulse until a paste forms (or use a large bowl and a handheld immersion blender).

2. Transfer the chickpea mixture to a bowl and add the couscous and eggs, mixing thoroughly to combine.

3. Chill the mixture in the refrigerator for 1 hour to firm it.

4. Form the couscous mixture into 4 patties.

5. Place a large skillet over medium-high heat and add the olive oil.

6. Place the patties in the skillet, 2 at a time, gently pressing them down with the back of a spatula. Cook for 5 minutes or until golden, and flip the patties over.

7. Cook the other side for 5 minutes and transfer the cooked burgers to a plate covered with a paper towel.

8. Repeat with the remaining 2 burgers.

PER SERVING Calories: 242; Fat: 10g; Carbohydrates: 29g; Phosphorus: 108mg;

Potassium: 168mg; Sodium: 43mg; Protein: 9g

MARINATED TOFU STIR-FRY

Serves 4 Prep time: 20 minutes, plus 2 hours chilling time; Cook time: 20 minutes

Tofu is an incredible ingredient that soaks up any flavors. It is a good source of protein and excellent source of calcium. Tofu is sold in different textures, from silken to extra-firm, so it can be used in many types of cuisine. Extra-firm tofu is best when you are marinating and stir-frying because it will hold its shape and not fall apart.

Ingredients
FOR THE TOFU
1 tablespoon freshly squeezed lemon juice
1 teaspoon minced garlic
1 teaspoon grated fresh ginger
Pinch red pepper flakes
5 ounces extra-firm tofu, pressed well and cubed (see ingredient tip)

FOR THE STIR-FRY

1 tablespoon olive oil
½ cup cauliflower florets
½ cup thinly sliced carrots
½ cup julienned red pepper
½ cup fresh green beans
2 cups cooked white rice

Directions

TO MAKE THE TOFU

1. In a small bowl, mix together the lemon juice, garlic, ginger, and red pepper flakes.
2. Add the tofu and toss to coat.
3. Place the bowl in the refrigerator and marinate for 2 hours.

TO MAKE THE STIR FRY

1. In a large skillet over medium-high heat, heat the oil.
2. Sauté the tofu for about 8 minutes or until it is lightly browned and heated through.
3. Add the cauliflower and carrots and sauté for 5 minutes, stirring and tossing Constantly.
4. Add the red pepper and green beans; sauté for 3 additional minutes.
5. Serve over the white rice.

Ingredient tip: Draining tofu is a crucial step to ensure this porous product absorbs all the flavor in the dish. Place the tofu on a paper towel-lined plate and cover the block with more paper towels. Set something heavy such as a large can or a book on the tofu. Check the drainage every 30 minutes, changing the paper towels if needed, for two hours.

Dialysis modification: Omit the red peppers from the dish to lower the amount of potassium in the recipe.

PER SERVING Calories: 190; Fat: 6g; Carbohydrates: 30g; Phosphorus: 90mg; Potassium: 199mg; Sodium: 22mg; Protein: 6g

THAI-INSPIRED VEGETABLE CURRY

Serves 4 Prep time: 15 minutes; Cook time: 45 minutes

Curry is a versatile dish that is equally at home in a fine-dining restaurant or eaten from a takeout box. This is because curry spices combine beautifully with many different ingredients, such as the eggplant, peppers, and carrots in this recipe. If you prefer a creamier sauce, add ¼ cup heavy (whipping) cream right at the end.

Ingredients
2 teaspoons olive oil
½ sweet onion, diced
2 teaspoons minced garlic
2 teaspoons grated fresh ginger
½ eggplant, peeled and diced
1 carrot, peeled and diced
1 red bell pepper, diced
1 tablespoon Hot Curry Powder (here)
1 teaspoon ground cumin
½ teaspoon coriander

Pinch cayenne pepper

1½ cups homemade vegetable stock

1 tablespoon cornstarch

¼ cup water

Directions

1. In a large stockpot over medium-high heat, heat the oil.

2. Sauté the onion, garlic, and ginger for 3 minutes or until they are softened.

3. Add the eggplant, carrots, and red pepper, and sauté, stirring often, for 6 additional minutes.

4. Stir in the curry powder, cumin, coriander, cayenne pepper, and vegetable stock.

5. Bring the curry to a boil and then reduce the heat to low.

6. Simmer the curry for about 30 minutes or until the vegetables are tender.

7. In a small bowl, stir together the cornstarch and water.

8. Stir the cornstarch mixture into the curry and simmer for about 5 minutes or until the sauce is thickened.

PER SERVING Calories: 100; Fat: 3g; Carbohydrates: 9g; Phosphorus: 28mg; Potassium: 180mg; Sodium: 218mg; Protein: 1g

LINGUINE WITH ROASTED RED PEPPER– BASIL SAUCE

Serves 4 Prep time: 20 minutes; Cook time: 20 minutes

Fresh basil imparts a wonderful aroma and flavor to this simple dish. a popular opinion is that herb's oils and extracts have antioxidant and antibacterial properties. Two of the vitamins it offers are vitamin A and blood-clotting vitamin
K. When cooking with basil, add it to the dish at the end to retain the best color and maximum flavor.

Ingredients

8 ounces uncooked linguine
1 teaspoon olive oil
½ sweet onion, chopped
2 teaspoons minced garlic
1 cup chopped roasted red bell peppers
1 teaspoon balsamic vinegar
¼ cup shredded fresh basil
Pinch red pepper flakes
Freshly ground black pepper

4 teaspoons grated low-fat Parmesan cheese, for garnish

Directions

1. Cook the pasta according to the package instructions.

2. While the pasta is cooking, place a large skillet over medium-high heat and add the olive oil.

3. Sauté the onions and garlic for about 3 minutes or until they are softened.

4. Add the red pepper, vinegar, basil, and red pepper flakes to the skillet and stir for about 5 minutes or until heated through.

5. Toss the cooked pasta with the sauce and season with pepper.

6. Serve topped with Parmesan cheese.

PER SERVING Calories: 246; Fat: 3g; Carbohydrates: 41g; Phosphorus: 117mg; Potassium: 187mg; Sodium: 450mg; Protein: 13g

BAKED MAC AND CHEESE

Serves 4 Prep time: 10 minutes; Cook time: 25 minutes

Creamy, rich, and cheesy is an accurate description of macaroni and cheese, but it doesn't have to be a guilty indulgence. This version has a hint of cayenne pepper, mustard, and garlic in the sauce, which adds a little heat in the background. Eat it immediately after cooking, because the sauce will become grainy if frozen and reheated.

Ingredients

Butter, for greasing the baking dish
1 teaspoon olive oil
½ sweet onion, chopped
1 teaspoon minced garlic
¼ cup rice milk
1 cup cream cheese
½ teaspoon dry mustard
½ teaspoon freshly ground black pepper
Pinch cayenne pepper
3 cups cooked macaroni

Directions

1. Preheat the oven to 375°F.

2. Grease a 9-by-9-inch baking dish with butter; set aside.

3. In a medium saucepan over medium heat, heat the olive oil.

4. Sauté the onion and garlic for about 3 minutes or until softened.

5. Stir in the milk, cheese, mustard, black pepper, and cayenne pepper until the mixture is smooth and well blended.

6. Add the cooked macaroni, stirring to coat.

7. Spoon the mixture into the baking dish and place in the oven.

8. Bake for about 15 minutes or until the macaroni is bubbly.

Dialysis modification: This dish is rich, so you can choose a smaller portion size to reduce your phosphorus and potassium intake.

PER SERVING Calories: 386; Fat: 22g; Carbohydrates: 37g; Phosphorus: 120mg;

Potassium: 146mg; Sodium: 219mg; Protein: 10g

GRILLED KALE AND FRIED EGG ON BREAD

Serves 2 Prep time: 10 minutes; Cook time: 20 minutes

A simple egg on a piece of toast becomes extraordinary with the addition of oven-crisped kale. This healthy green is packed with protein, fiber, and vitamins A, C, and K. It even offers some heart-healthy omega-3 fatty acids. When you buy kale at the supermarket, choose a bunch with dark, crisp leaves. When you cook with it, remove the ribs and toughest leaves first.

Ingredients
2 medium kale leaves
½ teaspoon olive oil
Pinch red pepper flakes
4 teaspoons unsalted butter, divided
2 slices white bread
2 teaspoons cream cheese
2 small eggs
Freshly ground black pepper

Directions

1. Preheat the oven to 350°F.

2. Massage the kale leaves with the olive oil until they are completely coated.

3. Sprinkle a pinch of red pepper flakes over the kale leaves.

4. Place the leaves in a pie plate and roast for about 10 minutes or until crispy.

5. Remove the kale from the oven; set aside.

6. Butter both sides of the bread with 1 teaspoon butter per slice.

7. In a large skillet over medium-high heat, toast the bread on both sides for about 3 minutes or until it is golden brown.

8. Remove the bread from the skillet and spread 1 teaspoon cream cheese on each slice.

9. Melt the remaining 2 teaspoons of butter in the skillet and fry the eggs sunny-side up, for about 4 minutes.

10. Place a piece of crispy kale and a fried egg on top of each slice of the cream cheese–topped bread.

11. Serve seasoned with pepper.

PER SERVING Calories: 224; Fat: 15g; Carbohydrates: 14g; Phosphorus: 118mg; Potassium: 175mg; Sodium: 200mg; Protein: 8g

TOFU AND EGGPLANT STIR-FRY

Serves 4 Prep time: 20 minutes; Cook time: 20 minutes

Garlic, jalapeño, and ginger contribute to the intense flavor of the sauce in this recipe. Garlic reduce the risk of heart disease and high blood pressure. It may also protect against some cancers, fight inflammation, and give your immune system a boost. This recipe is delicious when served over rice or noodles.

ingredients

1 tablespoon granulated sugar
1 tablespoon all-purpose flour
1 teaspoon grated fresh ginger
1 teaspoon minced garlic
1 teaspoon minced jalapeño pepper
Juice of 1 lime
Water
2 tablespoons olive oil, divided

5 ounces extra-firm tofu, cut into ½-inch cubes

2 cups cubed eggplant

2 scallions, both green and white parts, sliced

3 tablespoons chopped cilantro

Directions

1. In a small bowl, whisk together the sugar, flour, ginger, garlic, jalapeño, lime juice, and enough water to make ⅔ cup of sauce; set aside.

2. In a large skillet over medium-high heat, heat 1 tablespoon of the oil.

3. Sauté the tofu for about 6 minutes or until it is crisp and golden.

4. Remove the tofu; set aside on a plate.

5. Add the remaining 1 tablespoon oil and sauté the eggplant cubes for about 10 minutes or until they are fully cooked and lightly browned.

6. Add the tofu and scallions to the skillet and toss to combine.

7. Pour in the sauce and bring to a boil, stirring constantly, for about 2 minutes or until the sauce is thickened.

8. Add the cilantro before serving.

PER SERVING Calories: 386; Fat: 22g; Carbohydrates: 37g; Phosphorus: 120mg;

Potassium: 146mg; Sodium: 219mg; Protein: 10g

MIE GORENG WITH BROCCOLI

Serves 4 Prep time: 10 minutes, plus 30 minutes draining time; Cook time: 20 minutes

Indonesian food has complex flavors that stimulate the taste buds with salty, sweet, bitter, and spicy all at the same time. This dish includes sambal oelek, a spicy chile sauce from Southeast Asia. The word sambal is Indonesian for a sauce made with green chiles, and oelek refers to the technique to make it using a mortar and pestle.

Ingredients
½ pound rice noodles
¼ cup packed dark brown sugar
2 teaspoons minced garlic
1 teaspoon grated fresh ginger
1 teaspoon low-sodium soy sauce
½ teaspoon sambal oelek
4 ounces extra-firm tofu, cut into ½-inch cubes

1 tablespoon cornstarch

2 tablespoons olive oil, divided

2 cups broccoli, cut into small florets

2 scallions, both green and white parts, sliced thin on the diagonal Lime wedges, for garnish

Directions

1. Cook the noodles according to the package instructions; drain and set aside.

2. In a small bowl, whisk together the brown sugar, garlic, ginger, soy sauce, and sambal oelek; set aside.

3. Drain the tofu on paper towels for 30 minutes and pat the tofu dry.

4. Toss the tofu with the cornstarch and shake to remove the excess.

5. In a large skillet over medium-high heat, heat 1 tablespoon of the olive oil.

6. Add the tofu and sauté for about 10 minutes or until the tofu is browned on all sides and crispy.

7. Transfer the tofu to a plate with a slotted spoon.

8. Add the remaining 1 tablespoon oil to the skillet.

9. Sauté the broccoli for about 4 minutes or until it is tender.

10. Add the sauce and tofu to the skillet and cook for about 2 minutes or until the sauce thickens.

11. Serve topped with scallions and garnish with lime wedges.

PER SERVING Calories: 360; Fat: 11g; Carbohydrates: 62g; Phosphorus: 120mg; Potassium: 193mg; Sodium: 166mg; Protein: 4g

DESSERTS RECIPES

TART APPLE GRANITA

Serves 4 / Prep time: 15 minutes, plus 4 hours freezing time

Granita has a pleasing texture from the large ice crystals that form when the liquid freezes. For a more intense apple flavor, you can try fresh apple juice instead of using prepared juice from a can or bottle. Granny Smith, McIntosh, or Spartan apples are the best choices for a truly tart iced treat.

Ingredients
½ cup granulated sugar
½ cup water
2 cups unsweetened apple juice
¼ cup freshly squeezed lemon juice

Directions
1. In a small saucepan over medium-high heat, heat the sugar and water.
2. Bring the mixture to a boil and then reduce the heat to low and simmer for about 15 minutes or until the liquid has reduced by half.

3. Remove the pan from the heat and pour the liquid into a large shallow metal pan.

4. Let the liquid cool for about 30 minutes and then stir in the apple juice and lemon juice.

5. Place the pan in the freezer.

6. After 1 hour, run a fork through the liquid to break up any ice crystals that have formed. Scrape down the sides as well.

7. Place the pan back in the freezer and repeat the stirring and scraping every 20 minutes, creating slush.

8. Serve when the mixture is completely frozen and looks like crushed ice, after about 3 hours.

PER SERVING Calories: 157; Fat: 0g; Carbohydrates: 0g; Phosphorus: 10mg; Potassium: 141mg; Sodium: 5mg; Protein: 0g

LEMON-LIME SHERBET

Serves 8 Prep time: 5 minutes, plus 3 hours chilling time; Cook time: 15 minutes

Sherbet is the creamier version of sorbet. A little cream or milk is added to what is essentially a sorbet mixture, and the result is a frozen dessert that's richer than sorbet but lighter than ice cream. This sherbet has heavy cream as its dairy component and is a nice, tart choice for a refreshing summertime dessert. Top a bowl of this sherbet with fresh mint sprigs and a sprinkle of toasted coconut for a special finish.

Ingredients

2 cups water
1 cup granulated sugar
3 tablespoons lemon zest, divided
½ cup freshly squeezed lemon juice
Zest of 1 lime
Juice of 1 lime
½ cup heavy (whipping) cream

Directions

1. Place a large saucepan over medium-high heat and add the water, sugar, and 2 tablespoons of the lemon zest.

2. Bring the mixture to a boil and then reduce the heat and simmer for 15 minutes.

3. Transfer the mixture to a large bowl and add the remaining 1 tablespoon lemon zest, the lemon juice, lime zest, and lime juice.

4. Chill the mixture in the fridge until completely cold, about 3 hours.

5. Whisk in the heavy cream and transfer the mixture to an ice cream maker.

6. Freeze according to the manufacturer's instructions.

PER SERVING Calories: 151; Fat: 6g; Carbohydrates: 26g; Phosphorus: 10mg; Potassium: 27mg; Sodium: 6mg; Protein: 0g

TROPICAL VANILLA SNOW CONE

Serves 4 / Prep time: 15 minutes, plus freezing time

The best way to serve this sweet, pale pink treat is in old-fashioned pointed paper cups to mimic the look of a real snow cone. If you want to save time creating the icy texture, pop the entire frozen-fruit mixture out of the dish and pulse it in a food processor until it resembles snow. This will only work if you are serving the dessert right away and you eat all of it in one sitting.

Ingredients
1 cup canned peaches
1 cup pineapple
1 cup frozen strawberries
6 tablespoons water
2 tablespoons granulated sugar
1 tablespoon vanilla extract

Directions

1. In a large saucepan, mix together the peaches, pineapple, strawberries, water, and sugar over medium-high heat and bring to a boil.

2. Reduce the heat to low and simmer the mixture, stirring occasionally, for 15 minutes.

3. Remove from the heat and let the mixture cool completely, for about 1 hour.

4. Stir in the vanilla and transfer the fruit mixture to a food processor or blender.

5. Purée until smooth, and pour the purée into a 9-by-13-inch glass baking dish.

6. Cover and place the dish in the freezer overnight.

7. When the fruit mixture is completely frozen, use a fork to scrape the sorbet until you have flaked flavored ice.

8. Scoop the ice flakes into 4 serving dishes.

PER SERVING Calories: 92; Fat: 0g; Carbohydrates: 22g; Phosphorus: 17mg; Potassium: 145mg; Sodium: 4mg; Protein: 1g

PAVLOVA WITH PEACHES

Serves 8 Prep time: 30 minutes; Cook time: 1 hour, plus cooling time

Pavlovas are a simple, baked meringue topped with fruit, chocolate, or sauces. Meringue is not difficult to make, but some simple tricks will ensure success.

Separate the eggs when they are cold, so the yolks are less likely to break. Even the slightest hint of yolk in the whites can impede the beating process. Crack the eggs individually over a glass and then transfer the white into a bowl, so only one egg white will be ruined if the yolk breaks.

Ingredients

4 large egg whites, at room temperature
½ teaspoon cream of tartar
1 cup superfine sugar
½ teaspoon pure vanilla extract
2 cups drained canned peaches in juice

Directions

1. Preheat the oven to 225°F.
2. Line a baking sheet with parchment paper; set aside.

3. In a large bowl, beat the egg whites for about 1 minute or until soft peaks form.

4. Beat in the cream of tartar.

5. Add the sugar, 1 tablespoon at a time, until the egg whites are very stiff and glossy. Do not overbeat.

6. Beat in the vanilla.

7. Evenly spoon the meringue onto the baking sheet so that you have 8 rounds.

8. Use the back of the spoon to create an indentation in the middle of each round.

9. Bake the meringues for about 1 hour or until a light brown crust forms.

10. Turn off the oven and let the meringues stand, still in the oven, overnight.

11. Remove the meringues from the sheet and place them on serving plates.

12. Spoon the peaches, dividing evenly, into the centers of the meringues, and serve.

13. Store any unused meringues in a sealed container at room temperature for up to 1 week.

PER SERVING Calories: 132; Fat: 0g; Carbohydrates: 32g; Phosphorus: 7mg; Potassium: 95mg; Sodium: 30mg; Protein: 2g

BAKED PEACHES WITH CREAM CHEESE

Serves 4 Prep time: 10 minutes; Cook time: 15 minutes

Canned peaches become an elegant, rich dessert when stuffed with sweet, crunchy cookie crumbles, tart cream cheese, and honey. Peaches packed in juice, water, or light syrup are the best choice for this recipe. Peaches are an excellent source of fiber and vitamins A and C.

Ingredients

1 cup plain cream cheese, at room temperature

½ cup crushed Meringue Cookies (here)

¼ teaspoon ground cinnamon

Pinch ground nutmeg

8 canned peach halves, in juice

2 tablespoons honey

Directions

1. Preheat the oven to 350°F.

2. Line a baking sheet with parchment paper; set aside.

3. In a small bowl, stir together the cream cheese, meringue cookies, cinnamon, and nutmeg.

4. Spoon the cream cheese mixture evenly into the cavities in the peach halves.

5. Place the peaches on the baking sheet and bake for about 15 minutes or until the fruit is soft and the cheese is melted.

6. Remove the peaches from the baking sheet onto plates, 2 per person, and drizzle with honey before serving.

PER SERVING Calories: 260; Fat: 20g; Carbohydrates: 19g; Phosphorus: 74mg; Potassium: 198mg; Sodium: 216mg; Protein: 4g

SWEET CINNAMON CUSTARD

Serves 6 Prep time: 20 minutes, plus 1 hour chilling time; Cook time: 1 hour

Baked custards are cool and creamy with a velvety smoothness. A moist cooking environment is essential to avoid curdling the custard mixture like scrambled eggs, so always remember the water-bath step. Try adding carob powder, fruit purée, coffee, and other flavoring extracts for unique variations of this basic custard recipe.

Ingredients

Unsalted butter, for greasing the ramekins
1½ cups plain rice milk
4 eggs
¼ cup granulated sugar
1 teaspoon pure vanilla extract
½ teaspoon ground cinnamon Cinnamon sticks, for garnish (optional)

Directions

1. Preheat the oven to 325°F.
2. Lightly grease 6 (4-ounce) ramekins and place them in a baking dish; set aside.

3. In a large bowl, whisk together the rice milk, eggs, sugar, vanilla, and cinnamon until the mixture is very smooth.

4. Pour the mixture through a fine sieve into a pitcher.

5. Evenly divide the custard mixture among the ramekins.

6. Fill the baking dish with hot water, taking care not to get any water in the ramekins, until the water reaches halfway up the sides of the ramekins.

7. Bake for about 1 hour or until the custards are set and a knife inserted in the center of one of the custards comes out clean.

8. Remove the custards from the oven and take the ramekins out of the water.

9. Cool on wire racks for 1 hour and then transfer the custards to the refrigerator to chill for an additional hour.

10. Garnish each custard with a cinnamon stick, if desired.

PER SERVING Calories: 110; Fat: 4g; Carbohydrates: 14g; Phosphorus: 100mg; Potassium: 64mg; Sodium: 71mg; Protein: 4g

RASPBERRY BRÛLÉE

Serves 4 Prep time: 15 minutes; Cook time: 1 minute

This dessert is not the crème brûlée you might have eaten in high-end restaurants. You will not need to fiddle with water baths to create the smooth, tart base of this dessert; it is unbaked and simple. The burned sugar or brûlée happens in the oven, but if you want to create the crackly, caramelized sugar crust like a professional chef, use a handheld kitchen torch on each ramekin.

Ingredients

½ cup light sour cream
½ cup plain cream cheese, at room temperature
¼ cup brown sugar, divided
¼ teaspoon ground cinnamon
1 cup fresh raspberries

Directions

1. Preheat the oven to broil.

2. In a small bowl, beat together the sour cream, cream cheese, 2 tablespoons brown sugar, and cinnamon for about 4 minutes or until the mixture is very smooth and fluffy.

3. Evenly divide the raspberries among 4 (4-ounce) ramekins.

4. Spoon the cream cheese mixture over the berries and smooth the tops.

5. Store the ramekins in the refrigerator, covered, until you are ready to serve the dessert.

6. Sprinkle ½ tablespoon brown sugar evenly over each ramekin.

7. Place the ramekins on a baking sheet and broil 4 inches from the heating element until the sugar is caramelized and golden brown.

8. Remove from the oven. Let the brûlées sit 1 minute, and serve.

PER SERVING Calories: 188; Fat: 13g; Carbohydrates: 16g; Phosphorus: 60mg; Potassium: 158mg; Sodium: 132mg; Protein: 3g

VANILLA-INFUSED COUSCOUS PUDDING

Serves 6 Prep time: 20 minutes; Cook time: 20 minutes

Couscous replaces rice in this dish, creating a slightly different taste and a unique texture. The vanilla bean adds superior flavor to the pudding, but you can substitute extract if you do not have beans. Look for whole vanilla beans in the baking section of your local grocery store.

Ingredients

1½ cups plain rice milk
½ cup water
1 vanilla bean, split
½ cup honey
¼ teaspoon ground cinnamon
1 cup couscous

Directions

1. In a large saucepan, mix together the rice milk, water, and vanilla bean in large saucepan over medium heat.

2. Bring the milk to a gentle simmer, reduce the heat to low, and let the milk simmer for

10 minutes to allow the vanilla flavor to infuse into the milk.

3. Remove the saucepan from the heat.

4. Take out the vanilla bean and, using the tip of a paring knife, scrape the seeds from the pod into the warm milk.

5. Stir in the honey and cinnamon.

6. Stir in the couscous, cover the pan, and let it stand for 10 minutes.

7. With a fork, fluff the couscous before serving.

PER SERVING Calories: 334; Fat: 1g; Carbohydrates: 77g; Phosphorus: 119mg; Potassium: 118mg; Sodium: 41mg; Protein: 6g

HONEY BREAD PUDDING

**Serves 6 Prep time: 15 minutes, plus 3
hours soaking time; Cook time: 40
minutes**

This version of bread pudding is similar to
tender French toast sliced into large pieces.
The soft bread is infused with the egg and
milk mixture, creating a velvety custard and
a caramelized golden crust. Try topping this
dessert with an extra drizzle of honey and
fresh whipped cream.

Ingredients

Unsalted butter, for greasing the baking dish
1½ cups plain rice milk
2 eggs
2 large egg whites
¼ cup honey
1 teaspoon pure vanilla extract
6 cups cubed white bread

Directions

1. Lightly grease an 8-by-8-inch baking dish with butter; set aside.

2. In a medium bowl, whisk together the rice milk, eggs, egg whites, honey, and vanilla.

3. Add the bread cubes and stir until the bread is coated.

4. Transfer the mixture to the baking dish and cover with plastic wrap.

5. Store the dish in the refrigerator at least 3 hours.

6. Preheat the oven to 325°F.

7. Remove the plastic wrap from the baking dish and bake the pudding for 35 to 40 minutes or until golden brown and a knife inserted in the center comes out clean.

8. Serve warm.

PER SERVING Calories: 167; Fat: 3g; Carbohydrates: 30g; Phosphorus: 95mg; Potassium: 93mg; Sodium: 189mg; Protein: 6g

RHUBARB CRUMBLE

Serves 6 Prep time: 15 minutes; Cook time: 30 minutes

Fruit crumble belongs in a delicious dessert category that includes crisps, brown Betty, and cobblers. Crumbles usually do not contain nuts or oats, so the topping seems more like a butter cookie than a crust. Make this crumble with any kind of fruit, depending on the season and your personal preference.

Ingredients

Unsalted butter, for greasing the baking dish
1 cup all-purpose flour
½ cup brown sugar
½ teaspoon ground cinnamon
½ cup unsalted butter, at room temperature
1 cup chopped rhubarb
2 apples, peeled, cored, and sliced thin
2 tablespoons granulated sugar
2 tablespoons water

Directions

1. Preheat the oven to 325°F.

2. Lightly grease an 8-by-8-inch baking dish with butter; set aside.

3. In a small bowl, stir together the flour, sugar, and cinnamon until well combined.

4. Add the butter and rub the mixture between your fingers until it resembles coarse crumbs.

5. In a medium saucepan, mix together the rhubarb, apple, sugar, and water over medium heat and cook for about 20 minutes or until the rhubarb is soft.

6. Spoon the fruit mixture into the baking dish and evenly top with the crumble.

7. Bake the crumble for 20 to 30 minutes or until golden brown.

8. Serve hot.

PER SERVING Calories: 450; Fat: 23g; Carbohydrates: 60g; Phosphorus: 51mg; Potassium: 181mg; Sodium: 10mg; Protein: 4g

GINGERBREAD LOAF

Serves 16 Prep time: 20 minutes; Cook time: 1 hour

Fragrant spices and a hint of sweetness make gingerbread a perfect choice for dessert any time of the year. The distinct flavor comes from the addition of fresh ginger. If you want to use ground ginger instead, add 1 tablespoon with the dry ingredients.

Ingredients

Unsalted butter, for greasing the baking dish
3 cups all-purpose flour
½ teaspoon Ener-G baking soda substitute
2 teaspoons ground cinnamon
1 teaspoon ground allspice
¾ cup granulated sugar
1¼ cups plain rice milk
1 large egg
¼ cup olive oil
2 tablespoons molasses
2 teaspoons grated fresh ginger Powdered sugar, for dusting

Directions

1. Preheat the oven to 350°F,

2. Lightly grease a 9-by-13-inch baking dish with butter; set aside.

3. In a large bowl, sift together the flour, baking soda substitute, cinnamon, and allspice.

4. Stir the sugar into the flour mixture.

5. In medium bowl, whisk together the milk, egg, olive oil, molasses, and ginger until well blended.

6. Make a well in the center of the flour mixture and pour in the wet ingredients.

7. Mix until just combined, taking care not to overmix.

8. Pour the batter into the baking dish and bake for about 1 hour or until a wooden pick inserted in the middle comes out clean.

9. Serve warm with a dusting of powdered sugar.

PER SERVING Calories: 232; Fat: 5g; Carbohydrates: 42g; Phosphorus: 54mg; Potassium: 104mg; Sodium: 18mg; Protein: 4g

ELEGANT LAVENDER COOKIES

**Makes 24 cookies Prep time: 10 minutes;
Cook time: 15 minutes**

There are more than 30 varieties of lavender,
which can be grown in almost any area of
the world with success. Lavender is not
typically used in cooking, although it is
edible and combines very well with many
taste profiles. Lavender lends itself best to
delicate desserts and baked items such as
these elegant, buttery cookies.

Ingredients

5 dried organic lavender flowers, the entire
top of the flower
½ cup granulated sugar
1 cup unsalted butter, at room temperature
2 cups all-purpose flour
1 cup rice flour

Directions

1. Strip the tiny lavender flowers off the main stem carefully and place the flowers and granulated sugar into a food processor or blender. Pulse until the mixture is finely chopped.

2. In a medium bowl, cream together the butter and lavender sugar until it is very fluffy.

3. Mix the flours into the creamed mixture until the mixture resembles fine crumbs.

4. Gather the dough together into a ball and then roll it into a long log.

5. Wrap the cookie dough in plastic and refrigerate it for about 1 hour or until firm.

6. Preheat the oven to 375°F.

7. Slice the chilled dough into ¼-inch rounds and refrigerate it for 1 hour or until firm.

8. Bake the cookies for 15 to 18 minutes or until they are a very pale, golden brown.

9. Let the cookies cool.

10. Store the cookies at room temperature in a sealed container for up to 1 week.

PER SERVING Calories: 153; Fat: 9g; Carbohydrates: 17g; Phosphorus: 18mg; Potassium: 17mg; Sodium: 0mg; Protein: 1g

CAROB ANGEL FOOD CAKE

Serves 16 Prep time: 30 minutes; Cook time: 30 minutes

Angel food cake is a favorite of many people, especially in the summer months. Carob is a delicious substitution for cocoa powder that is lower in fat and higher in carbohydrates. This angel food cake would be fantastic paired with a cascade of fresh raspberries and topped with a dollop of whipped cream.

Ingredients
¾ cup all-purpose flour
¼ cup carob flour
1½ cups sugar, divided
12 large egg whites, at room temperature
1½ teaspoons cream of tartar
2 teaspoons vanilla

Directions
1. Preheat the oven to 375°F.
2. In a medium bowl, sift together the all-purpose flour, carob flour, and ¾ cup of the sugar; set aside.

3. Beat the egg whites and cream of tartar with a hand mixer for about 5 minutes or until soft peaks form.

4. Add the remaining ¾ cup sugar by the tablespoon to the egg whites until all the sugar is used up and stiff peaks form.

5. Fold in the flour mixture and vanilla.

6. Spoon the batter into an angel food cake pan.

7. Run a knife through the batter to remove any air pockets.

8. Bake the cake for about 30 minutes or until the top springs back when pressed lightly.

9. Invert the pan onto a wire rack to cool.

10. Run a knife around the rim of the cake pan and remove the cake from the pan.

PER SERVING Calories: 113; Fat: 0g; Carbohydrates: 25g; Phosphorus: 11mg; Potassium: 108mg; Sodium: 42mg; Protein: 3g

OLD-FASHIONED APPLE KUCHEN

Serves 16 Prep time: 25 minutes; Cook time: 1 hour

Apfel kuchen means "apple cake" in German. This version is a simple spiced cake studded with apples and served warm. Plums, peaches, pears, and berries can be substituted easily for the apples.

Ingredients

Unsalted butter, for greasing the baking dish
1 cup unsalted butter, at room temperature
2 cups granulated sugar
2 eggs, beaten
2 teaspoons pure vanilla extract
2 cups all-purpose flour
1 teaspoon Ener-G baking soda substitute
2 teaspoons ground cinnamon
½ teaspoon ground nutmeg
Pinch ground allspice
2 large apples, peeled, cored, and diced (about 3 cups)

Directions

1. Preheat the oven to 350°F.

2. Grease a 9-by-13-inch glass baking dish; set aside.

3. Cream together the butter and sugar with a hand mixer until light and fluffy, for about 3 minutes.

4. Add the eggs and vanilla and beat until combined, scraping down the sides of the bowl, about 1 minute.

5. In a small bowl, stir together the flour, baking soda substitute, cinnamon, nutmeg, and allspice.

6. Add the dry ingredients to the wet ingredients and stir to combine.

7. Stir in the apple and spoon the batter into the baking dish.

8. Bake for about 1 hour or until the cake is golden.

9. Cool the cake on a wire rack.

10. Serve warm or chilled.

PER SERVING Calories: 368; Fat: 16g; Carbohydrates: 53g; Phosphorus: 46mg; Potassium: 68mg; Sodium: 15mg; Protein: 3

BUTTERY POUND CAKE

Serves 20 Prep time: 20 minutes; Cook time: 1 hour, 15 minutes

Pound cake originated in Northern Europe. It got its name from the 1-pound measurements used for the ingredients—flour, butter, sugar, and eggs.

Cookbook measurements have since changed to cups, grams, and whole eggs, so the pound amounts are not as easy to notice. Over time, the original recipe also has evolved to include other ingredients such as sour cream, milk, baking soda, baking powder, and extracts for flavoring.

Ingredients

Unsalted butter, for greasing the baking pan
All-purpose flour, for dusting the baking pan
2 cups unsalted butter, at room temperature
3 cups granulated sugar
6 eggs, at room temperature
1 tablespoon pure vanilla extract
4 cups all-purpose flour
¾ cup unsweetened rice milk

Directions

1. Preheat the oven to 325°F.

2. Grease a 10-inch Bundt pan with butter and dust with flour; set aside.

3. In a large bowl, beat the butter and sugar with a hand mixer for about 4 minutes or until very fluffy and pale.

4. Add the eggs, one at a time, beating well after each addition and scraping down the sides of the bowl.

5. Beat in the vanilla.

6. Add the flour and rice milk, alternating in 3 additions, with the flour first and last.

7. Spoon the batter into the Bundt pan.

8. Bake for about 1 hour and 15 minutes or until the top of the cake is golden brown and the cake springs back when lightly pressed.

9. Cool the cake in the Bundt pan on a wire rack for 10 minutes.

10. Remove the cake from the pan to a wire rack and cool completely before serving.

PER SERVING Calories: 389; Fat: 20g; Carbohydrates: 50g; Phosphorus: 67mg; Potassium: 57mg; Sodium: 28mg; Protein: 5g

CPSIA information can be obtained
at www.ICGtesting.com
Printed in the USA
LVHW050735121220
674004LV00011B/297